Thriving *with* HYPOTHYROIDISM

Thriving

with

HYPOTHYROIDISM

THE HOLISTIC GUIDE
*to Losing Weight, Keeping It Off,
and Living a Vibrant Life*

SUSAN TUCKER
ANNA AUSTIN

NEW YORK

LONDON • NASHVILLE • MELBOURNE • VANCOUVER

Thriving with HYPOTHYROIDISM
THE HOLISTIC GUIDE *to Losing Weight,*
Keeping It Off, and Living a Vibrant Life

Published in New York, New York, by Morgan James Publishing in partnership with Difference Press. Morgan James is a trademark of Morgan James, LLC. www.MorganJamesPublishing.com

The Morgan James Speakers Group can bring authors to your live event. For more information or to book an event visit The Morgan James Speakers Group at www.TheMorganJamesSpeakersGroup.com.

ISBN 978-1-64279-149-5 paperback
ISBN 978-1-64279-150-1 eBook
Library of Congress Control Number: 2018907326

Cover Design by:
Rachel Lopez
www.r2cdesign.com

Interior Design by:
Bonnie Bushman
The Whole Caboodle Graphic Design

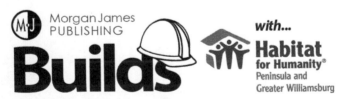

In an effort to support local communities, raise awareness and funds, Morgan James Publishing donates a percentage of all book sales for the life of each book to Habitat for Humanity Peninsula and Greater Williamsburg.

Get involved today! Visit
www.MorganJamesBuilds.com

We dedicate this book to the unconventional doctors and nurse practitioners who guided us along our health journey, who taught us to heal our thyroids by thinking outside the box and to let nutrition, exercise, and lifestyle changes be the cornerstones of our treatment.

Table of Contents

....

Introduction

....

"You must be the change you wish to see in the world."
– Gandhi

Why is it that we Americans are having such a love affair with prescription medicine? Don't misunderstand the question we are asking. In an acute situation, medicine is lifesaving or when the body has become so ill that it can't fight back on its own, medicine is absolutely life-giving. No question! But many drugs we take are simply masking the symptoms of disease and not curing the disease at all and maybe doing more harm than good.

It's the quick fix we are all after. We are too busy with being busy that we don't want to have to stop, take the time, and think about what we could do to prevent the disease in the first place or heal disease once it manifests. "The quick fix will work just fine, so why even bother" has become the mindset in today's society regarding health. We have heard so many times, *"They make a medicine for that and it's easier than watching what I eat, so I will take the medicine!"* As people age, they are usually on several prescriptions and changing their lifestyle or diet to be able to get off their medication is a scary proposition for them. They settle for the excuse that their disease comes with aging.

We should be asking the question, *"What is my responsibility in maintaining my health into old age?"* But sadly, taking the pill because it's easier in our fast-paced lives is the norm. Doing the work could mean giving up something that is pleasurable instead of trying to find a more suitable replacement. Most of us have been guilty of this at some time in our lives. We pop the ibuprofen for that headache instead of trying relaxation techniques or trying to determine why we have a headache in the first place. In many circles, ibuprofen is affectionately called vitamin I. We want that instant gratification and instant relief. We are not used to waiting. Healing takes time.

Did you know that over half of Americans are on prescription medication, taking four drugs, on average? We are taking more drugs today than ever before in history and far more than any other nation, and yet, we are sicker. Estimates from the Centers for Disease Control and Prevention say almost 1.3 million people in the U.S. went to hospital emergency rooms due to adverse drug interactions in 2014 and about 124,000 of those people died. What are these chemicals doing to our bodies? What kind of chemical soup is created in our blood when we mix several drugs together? What happens when we mix them with other chemicals we are coming in contact with? Can the mixture be causing damage to the body? Why has there been such an increase in the use of medications? Instead, we should be asking the question, *"What is the root cause of disease?"*

According to Medical News Today, the top leading cause of death in this country is still heart disease. What could prevent most of the heart disease in this country? A change in diet and lifestyle can dramatically reduce your chances of developing heart disease. Why shouldn't this be the first line of defense against such a pervasive disease?

The second leading cause of death in this country is cancer. According to the World Cancer Research Fund, one third of all cancers are related to conditions like being overweight, obesity, inactivity (sedentary), and having a poor diet. What could prevent a third of all cancers? Changes to diet and lifestyle.

Respiratory diseases are the third leading cause of death, with chronic obstructive pulmonary disease (COPD) being the primary condition, but also include bronchitis, emphysema, and asthma. Key factors in developing respiratory diseases are tobacco smoke and air pollution in the home and workplace. What could help these conditions? Again, it's about changes to diet and lifestyle, as well as cleaning up the air inside your home.

Other leading causes of death include accidents (that would include adverse drug interactions), strokes, Alzheimer's disease (which is also called diabetes of the brain), and diabetes. What could help these conditions? You've got it—changes to diet and lifestyle.

In addition to diseases caused by our diet and lifestyle choices, we had better think about our health care system. Our health care costs are increasing faster than our rise in wages. The average worker now spends $5,714 for a family health insurance plan, while the deductibles having to be paid out before the plan kicks in are skyrocketing as well. Most employers now are having their employees pay some amount out of pocket for individual policies because the cost to employers is becoming burdensome.

What is spearheading the rise in premiums? Analysts say it is directly related to the cost of medical treatments and the rise in chronic illnesses and obesity. We're spending more time in the doctor's office than ever before. Were you aware that nearly half of the U.S. population has one or more chronic conditions such as asthma, heart disease, or diabetes? When you combine that with the aging population and the number of obese people in America, along with inflated medical spending, it's a recipe for disaster. We are not even including the lack of transparency in the true cost of care and escalating cost of pharmaceuticals.

Some have proposed to make the ones with certain chronic conditions pay more of the burden by raising their premiums to be able to lower the premiums of the ones without certain conditions. Should obese people pay more? What about smokers? What about our elderly citizens? Should they carry the burden? Is that fair? When will it end? When will Americans say enough is enough? Now, more than ever, it's time to take personal responsibility for our health. Your life and your pocketbook depend on it.

I love the quote from Dr. Andrew Weil: "I have argued for years that we do not have a health care system in America. We have a disease-management system—one that depends on ruinously expensive drugs and surgeries that treat health conditions after they manifest rather than giving our citizens simple diet, lifestyle, and therapeutic tools to keep them healthy." Wouldn't it be wonderful if we could implement a true health care system where doctors looked at the root cause of disease? Wouldn't it be wonderful if medical schools taught their doctors about natural approaches to healing instead of only focusing on the drugs that are designed for treating the symptoms of disease?

Many doctors' hands are tied. With the growing population and the growing number of people with disease, getting appointments to see your doctor has become a big problem. Many are in busy practices that schedule only 15-20 minutes for a visit. This has to be so frustrating for these doctors. How can you do a thorough health assessment in that short amount of time? With the uncertainties of our health care system, it's more important—now than ever—to take your health into your own hands.

If you are reading this book, you have been diagnosed with hypothyroidism, or at least think you may be suffering from a sluggish thyroid. You have the symptoms: gaining weight, the inability to lose weight, the inability to maintain any weight loss that you do manage to lose, the debilitating fatigue, the brain fog, the hair loss, digestive issues, depression, and on and on. Maybe you've been told that your thyroid test is normal, but you're not convinced and you are not satisfied with that answer, and you think, "If I can get my hands on some medicine," or "If my doctor would just increase my dose, all would be well." As you will see, there is more to the story.

Let's start a movement! A revolution to get healthy and to stay healthy. Let's explore ways to improve our health naturally so we can live into our golden years, living vibrantly instead of being crippled with disease. Let's start a revolution in ourselves, in our families, in our communities. There is a better way of living!

What we are going to talk about in this book are things that Anna and I have found to be useful in controlling our own hypothyroid symptoms and the things we use to help our bodies heal themselves. All of this comes from 20 years of research— going to different types of doctors, different types of testing, exploring different diets and workout programs, and trying out different kinds of supplements. We will discuss what we've done right and what we've done wrong. We've done the gamut, and we want to share what we have learned.

We want to be clear that this book is not intended to be an anti-pharmaceutical drug book even though we have talked about prescription drug use in this country. It is, however, a book about taking personal responsibility and a more proactive approach to our own health. Every single human body on this planet is unique; and the only way to advocate for yourself and your health, is to first, be your own detective and figure out how your body ticks. That's what we will help you determine.

It's important to note that what Anna and I are going to share is not intended to be a substitute for your doctor's recommendations. This should be a complementary approach that will help you feel your best and help stop the progression of the disease.

Let's get started!

CHAPTER 1

Ella

*"Keep your face to the sunshine
and you can never see the shadow."*
– Helen Keller

J want to introduce you to a beautiful lady named Ella. She grew up in a small town in the eastern part of North Carolina. She was the youngest of four, and the only girl. Her brothers were very protective and watched out for their little sister as good brothers do. In a town so small, everyone knew everyone! Sundays meant church and dinner with her family and cousins at her grandmother's house. The ladies of the family were excellent southern cooks and all brought their specialties to the table! There was always enough food to feed the town. Her grandmother would say, "If you leave hungry,

1

it's your own fault!" Ella loved her family and the time spent together was always full of laughter and great stories from the ones wiser.

In high school, Ella was always very athletic; she was a top runner on her track team and was on a competitive cheerleading team outside of school. You could always find Ella at the gym running on a treadmill or in an aerobics class, giving it her all.

Since she was so active, she never had to worry about her weight. Ella had, what she thought, was a fairly healthy diet, but she loved pizza night out with her friends and an occasional good scoop of ice cream from the local creamery. She didn't have to worry about counting calories or counting carbs; in fact, she didn't give it much thought at all.

Ella had the bubbliest personality and the beauty to match. Long, silky blonde hair was her trademark. She never met a stranger who didn't notice her and would light up any room she entered, putting others at ease with her genuine kindness. She was a people person. She was the kind of friend everyone would go to when they needed advice. She was the motivator, the encourager, the positive thinker, the one who was always giving of herself.

After high school graduation, Ella went off to college with several of her friends and majored in business. She was the typical college student; never missing a "thirsty Thursday" at her favorite hangout or tailgating at the football games. She was very busy with school, and she spent many hours in the library studying. She managed to hit the gym several times a week, but certainly not as much as she did in high school.

The food in the cafeteria was not the delicious home-cooked meals she was used to, but being a college student, who had time to cook? She and her friends packed on the typical Freshman 15 as it seemed to be a right of passage to gain weight in college. She remembered seeing college students that would come back home for one of the big football games or holidays and seeing how much weight they had gained and thinking that would never happen to her. But it did. She started skipping meals and trying to run more and clock a few more hours in at the gym to lose those stubborn pounds. She would lose some but those pounds would come right back. She lost those same 15 pounds over and over again. This had never happened to her before. She had never struggled.

Ella started dating Brian in her junior year. They met in one of their business classes, and then started bumping into each other around campus and decided to go out to dinner. They had so much in common. The same upbringing, the same dreams, the same goals. They really hit it off. He was so handsome; brown hair and the bluest eyes she had ever seen that could stare straight into her heart. He loved the gym as much as she did and they worked out together. He was muscular but had a little beer belly that made her feel a little more comfortable about her newly acquired self-consciousness and extra pounds.

They started talking about getting married nearing the end of their senior year, because they couldn't stand the thought of not being together. They decided that he would get a job and then she would look for one in the same area. Brian landed a great job in Tennessee as a pharmaceutical sales representative for a large drug company. He proposed to Ella and they moved away to Tennessee. Ella was able to get a job as a medical device sales representative in the same area. They soon got married and began their lives together. They were living the dream! They both had good jobs with good salaries and with the potential for growth. Life was good.

After four years of marriage and working up the career ladder, they felt like something was missing. They wanted a family. This was a part of their dream to have a big family like they both grew up with. They both wanted at least two, or possibly three children. They thought the time was right to have a baby in their lives.

After seven months of trying, they were finally expecting their first baby! Everyone was so excited! They couldn't wait for the baby to be born! At their gender reveal party they learned that the baby was be a boy! Brian was so happy, and Ella was excited that any other siblings would have a big brother to look after them just like she had. They fixed the nursery and decorated it with a jungle theme. There was so much fun in the preparation.

Ella had morning sickness during the early weeks and actually lost a few pounds, but her second trimester was great! Food had never tasted so good! She was trying to eat healthily, but pizza was her weakness! She craved it! She gained 40 pounds and had swelling in her legs. She didn't dare take her shoes off before bed because her feet would swell so much that she couldn't put them back on. The doctor told her to watch what she was eating and that he didn't want her to gain weight at the rate she was gaining as it could cause complications. No more pizza!

Three weeks before their baby boy was born Ella's blood pressure was elevated and her ankles were swollen, so the doctor told her to stop work immediately and get bed rest. She did just that. On December 10, Ella and Brian welcomed their new bundle of joy into this world one week before his due date! They named him Christopher! They were so excited to finally get to meet this little fella and bring him home into their lives. Their bond grew tighter with every passing day. Christopher was the apple of their eyes. With maternity leave quickly coming to an end, the thought of going back to work and leaving Christopher for someone else to look after was crushing Ella. No one could love and care for him the way she did. She and Brian decided that they would be fine on Brian's salary for the time being, so she resigned from her job.

A couple of months after Christopher was born, things started to change. Ella's fatigue was overwhelming. Every night when she went to bed, she longed to be able to sleep through the night like she did before Christopher was born. It was such a struggle to get up to feed the baby during the night and to be able to have the energy to make it through the next day. Doing this night after night after night, no words could describe the exhaustion Ella was feeling. She began to wonder if she was a good mother for longing for the days before the baby. Even when her mother would come to visit and take care of Christopher for her so she could sleep, she never felt rested.

In the beginning, Ella began to lose the 50 plus pounds of pregnancy weight, and thought breast feeding was a miracle! But after a couple of months, her weight started increasing. No matter what she did she couldn't stop the weight gain. One pound turned into two, and two turned into four. It seemed like she was gaining a pound or two a week. Ella's milk supply was decreasing so that she could not pump enough for Brian to be able to take over when he got home from work. She had thoughts of giving up on breast feeding because it seemed to be so much work for her, and her thoughts turned to guilt over not wanting to give her baby the best possible start.

Christopher did not nap very well, and there were days that Ella realized she hadn't eaten, taken a bath, or even changed out of her pajamas. Looking after the baby was more than a full-time job. How could she ever be able to look after two children? How were other mothers able to handle more than one child? She felt so alone.

When Ella went to her doctor to discuss her fatigue, weight gain, and her anxiety, he said it was normal for new mothers to be tired and struggle with pregnancy weight. He prescribed her some sleeping pills and an anti-depressant, and sent her on her way without really listening to her. When she talked with her mother about her fatigue, her mother said she went through the same thing and it was normal. It was a part of being a mother. Ella didn't feel like this was what a new mother went through. She felt like every part of her body was sick.

A year after Christopher was born, Ella's weight continued to climb. She was now almost 75 pounds overweight and as she looked at herself in the mirror, she hardly recognized herself anymore. How could things have gotten so out of control? Brian gave her the advice to just go to the gym and work out like she used to. She wanted to punch him in the nose. Why was it so easy for him to lose weight? Why did she struggle so? It didn't seem fair. Why couldn't she seem to get it together?

However, she took Brian's advice and pushed herself and went to the gym and ran on the treadmill. After weeks of doing this, her weight hardly budged. She started skipping meals to see if that would help, but it didn't. She would get so hungry that she would overeat at the next meal. Ella wondered if Brian found her attractive anymore. Would things ever be normal again? Her hair was falling out. Her joints hurt. Her cholesterol was high. She had digestive problems. She got every virus that came to town. She knew something was different. She had never had these problems before pregnancy. She was healthy.

Ella decided to take the time to go to another doctor and get a second opinion. Her new doctor decided to run a test on the thyroid to see if that was the problem. The test came back that Ella had hypothyroidism, and he prescribed her the synthetic thyroid replacement hormone, Synthroid. After a couple of weeks, her energy improved somewhat, but she was still experiencing all of the other symptoms. Three months, six months—and still no real improvement. She began to wonder if her life would always be like this from now on. Would she ever want to have another baby? She wondered why this had happened to her.

Ella is at a crossroads. If she doesn't get to the root of why she has hypothyroidism, then several things could happen. She may continue to have to increase her medication as more and more of her thyroid is destroyed. She may never lose the weight and keep it off, and then suffer from all of the illnesses obesity causes. She may develop other autoimmune diseases over time and have to take medication to combat those illnesses. Other body systems may be further compromised, and she may develop cardiovascular disease. Her fertility may be affected in the event that she and Brian one day decide to have another baby.

Ella may be afraid of doing the work to get to the root of the problem. Because it is work! She may be afraid that she will not get the support she needs from Brian. She has always trusted conventional medicine and might not be willing to try something new. Remember that insanity is doing the same thing over and over again and expecting different results.

Were you aware that postpartum hypothyroidism occurs in one in every 17 women in the U.S.? For most, this is the autoimmune form of thyroid disease called Hashimoto's disease. In some, the hypothyroid state continues for about a year, and then clears on its own—but may come back later in life or after another pregnancy. There is usually a hyperthyroid phase in the first month or two when there is initial weight loss and energy, but the hypothyroid phase follows, and in most, the normal state of the thyroid doesn't return. We will talk about other causes of hypothyroidism as we go through the book. Oftentimes, there is a trigger that initiates the disease.

The body has the innate ability to heal itself if given the proper environment. If Ella implements the strategies we are suggesting in this book, she will prevent the further destruction of her thyroid, and she will be able to lose weight and keep it off and have an energy-filled life. Will she be able to get off of her thyroid medication? Well, that remains to be seen. It will depend on how much of her thyroid has been destroyed. If she is able to get off of her medication, the things we suggest will help to keep hypothyroidism from coming back. The sooner these suggestions are implemented, the faster she will recover her life. One thing is for sure, her medication will work better, and she will have more thyroid hormone working for her—instead of against her. She will be able to increase her metabolism, lose the weight and keep it off, and have more energy to do the things she loves and to look after her amazing family. The time is now to make that decision.

CHAPTER 2

A Mother's Story

"Motherhood: all love begins and ends there."
– Robert Browning

We want to start by sharing our story from the beginning. Our sweet, sweet Anna was born on October 14, 1987, two weeks before her due date. My pregnancy was great and the delivery was drug free. It was a completely different experience from my pregnancy and birth of my first-born son. Anna was such an easy baby. She slept through the night at four weeks old. I was so thankful she did; having two children 22 months apart, I needed my sleep!

I did not breast feed with either of my children, choosing to formula feed instead. We were not as aware of the benefits of breast feeding back then and not many of my friends chose to nurse. After a few weeks on cow's milk formula, Anna developed stomach upsets, with colic-like symptoms. Her pediatrician switched her to a soy formula because he felt like she was sensitive to cow's milk. There was not much improvement.

She had esophageal reflux for the first six months. She would spit up volumes at least 10-15 times a day. Sometimes it even came out of her nose, causing her to lose her breath, which scared us both. Anna's pediatrician kept a close eye on her weight gain to make sure she was growing. Even though I stayed home with her and my son until Anna was ten months old, she caught every cold that came around. Her colds would turn into ear infections and bronchitis almost every time. She had walking pneumonia one time, but I was able to keep her at home instead of going to the hospital. She developed viral-induced asthma, and I remember having to sit outside in the cold air to help her breathe at night. We had to go to the doctor's office for breathing treatments and she had an asthma inhaler we could use at home during a cold.

She had chronic ear infections, so her pediatrician prescribed long-term antibiotics to try to clear them up but tubes were inevitable. So, at almost a year old, we had tubes put into her ears. Prior to the tubes, Anna wasn't really babbling, because she wasn't really hearing. When we brought her home from the hospital after surgery, she screamed when she heard the train go by or when we ran the vacuum cleaner. She was hearing well for the first time in many months. She began talking as well. Somehow we made it through the first two years.

Anna was a happy, active child who never walked anywhere! She was always galloping or running wherever she went. She was the only girl in the family for a while, and she could outrun any of the boys as a child. In the second and third grade, things began to change. She began to gain weight. She was moody. It was taking her a long time to get her homework done at night. She was tired and generally just didn't feel good. She was beginning to be teased about her weight by her classmates, and she came to me one day crying and asked me for help. As a mother, I felt her pain. I just wanted to make everything better.

I made an appointment with her pediatrician to discuss her weight gain and other issues she was having. He totally dismissed my concerns and me. He told me that she had to be "sneaking food," that children didn't gain weight without eating! He tested her cholesterol and it was high (a problem with untreated hypothyroidism, I would later learn) which further supported his idea that it was the food she was eating. I cooked dinner most nights and I packed my children's lunches every day. Eating out was a Friday night treat (and would usually include steak and cheese subs and a night watching television with the children. Not so healthy.) He suggested that she was exchanging food with her classmates at school and to have the teacher keep an eye out for that. No one else in the family was having problems. Her brother was fine. It didn't add up. He told me I just wanted a "perfect" child and I needed to accept her for who she was. "She would grow out of this," he said.

I was mortified! I had a "perfect" child! She was asking for my help, and I was coming to him in turn. But instead, he made me feel ashamed of bringing up the weight issue. I was hurt, and felt like a terrible mother. He was the only pediatrician in our rural area in eastern North Carolina, so I accepted his diagnosis that she would "grow out of it" and went home. But I knew in my heart of hearts that there was something out of kilter. But he was the doctor! Who was I to question him? I was brought up that you accepted what people in authority said, especially a doctor, without questioning and do as they say to do!

None of this made sense to me because Anna was very active during the day even though she would crash and burn in the late afternoon. She won the county athletic award for the most sit-ups in a minute in the third grade. At a parent-teacher conference when Anna was in fourth grade, her PE teacher made a comment to me that Anna was such an athlete but to look at her you would not think so. I remember that conversation like it was yesterday. She thought something wasn't quite right as well. I was still confused and didn't understand what was going on.

We moved to Winston Salem, North Carolina, when Anna was in the fifth grade in 1998. She joined the neighborhood swim team and would practice two hours every morning that summer. The coach would line up the junior Olympians on one relay team to ensure first place, and Anna would always be on the second relay team. Her relay team got together at one meet and decided that they were going to give it all that they had and they were going to beat the junior Olympian relay team. If they were going to win, they would have to swim harder than ever! They swam their hearts out that day! Anna was the third swimmer, and they needed to make up time. When she dove into the water, I was stunned! I had never seen anything like it! She looked as if she was swimming on top of the water! Two men from the other team that were standing beside me commented to each other, "Look at that girl swim!" She was pouring it on! When she got to the end of the pool, the last leg of the relay dove in! Anna was at the edge but couldn't pull herself out of the water. There was so much commotion her coach wasn't paying attention. I went over and took one look at her face and arms, and what I saw terrified me! Her muscles were twitching all over (another sign of untreated hypothyroidism). She said she felt sick and she couldn't pull herself up! I reached down and helped her out of the pool and got her a soda thinking maybe she needed a sugar boost. Well, they didn't beat their junior Olympian teammates; they came in second as usual, but this would be a turning point. We would begin to get some answers.

What I saw after her swim terrified me so that I knew something was wrong. I carried her to her new family doctor and explained what I had seen and about the other issues Anna was experiencing. Having hypothyroidism herself, she recognized Anna's symptoms and she immediately ran a thyroid test. I got a call from the doctor on a Saturday morning, and she said Anna was the most hypothyroid patient she had ever seen and she had never seen hypothyroidism in a child of her age. The doctor was afraid that based on her symptoms and her thyroid levels, Anna could slip into a coma. She wanted her to go to the hospital immediately to get bloodwork done and then to start her on the synthetic form of the thyroid hormone, Synthroid, immediately.

I felt relieved because as a mother I knew something was wrong. I also felt guilty for not following my instincts and speaking up for my little girl. I felt guilty for not making an appointment with another doctor to get a second opinion, even if I did have to drive to another city. But I was afraid they would tell me the same thing; that I was focusing on weight gain—so I did nothing. I didn't want to raise a daughter who was focused on body image. At the same time, I was concerned for her health but didn't have the voice to question her doctor. I felt like we were finally getting some answers to some of the problems she was suffering from, the weight gain with no increase in calories (or sneaking food), the mood swings, falling asleep after school and not being able to wake her up for at least two hours, taking forever to do homework and the inability to get going in the mornings, and that high cholesterol! It was all finally making sense.

Once Anna was diagnosed, I began to read everything I could get my hands on which was not much back in 1998! I was putting my biology degree to good use. Research! Research! Research! The books were so limited and any discussion of children with hypothyroidism was almost non-existent. Less than 3 percent of all hypothyroid patients were children. That is probably why it really never occurred to Anna's first pediatrician to test her thyroid. After diagnosis, Anna was referred to the best endocrinologist in Winston Salem. He assured us that when her TSH (thyroid stimulating hormone, the blood test conventional doctors used to determine the health of the thyroid—more on this later) was in the normal range, Anna's metabolism would be normal, like that of any other child! The drug would replace any missing thyroid hormone, and all of the symptoms that would be associated with hypothyroidism would go away. This was *not* the case!

We were referred to a couple of registered dieticians that could only refer to the USDA food pyramid as the proper way to get nutrition with recommendations of adding more whole wheat and dairy. Even when Anna's TSH tested in the "normal range," she could not lose the weight. Even when she was on the neighborhood swim team for three years, practicing two hours a day, she still couldn't lose any weight and still had symptoms of still being hypothyroid. She was on her middle school basketball team and the symptoms persisted. We felt helpless! We wanted answers to why this was happening! Not bandages!

The final straw came when we went to her endocrinologist for an appointment when Anna was in the seventh grade. In addition to still having all of her hypothyroid symptoms, especially concerning to her was still her inability to lose weight—and now other symptoms were appearing as well. She was having problems with severe constipation. Her doctor told her having a bowel movement once a week was normal for her and people made too much over bowel movements. When we made it to the parking lot after that appointment, Anna screamed and yelled, "That man is an idiot! Get me another doctor! I *refuse* to go to him again!" This was so out of character for her to lose her temper like this. But, it was another turning point for us.

As more and more information was coming out about thyroid disease, I became curious about natural medicine. What we were doing wasn't working. I was a little skeptical! I was very conventional, even attending pharmacy school before I changed my major to biology. I didn't give it a second thought to use antibiotics and Tylenol with both of my children when they were babies. They both drank soy formula because they couldn't tolerate cow's milk formula. I always did what my doctors told me to do. They were the authorities. My brother actually told me about a naturopathic doctor in Asheville, North Carolina that he had been to and was really impressed with him. I was surprised that there was a doctor of natural medicine so close.

I made Anna an appointment with his nurse practitioner in the summer before her eighth grade. We had never had an appointment like this! She spent so much time asking questions and listening to us, something that we never experienced in a conventional office. She ran different types of tests that had never been run before. We found out that Anna was high in heavy metals. She changed her Synthroid medication to a natural desiccated thyroid medication that was used for years prior to the synthetic form. She recommended a diet that finally allowed Anna to feel better and lose weight! We were finally onto something wonderful and healing for the first time! It was just the beginning!

When I was in my mid 40s, I too, was diagnosed with hypothyroidism. I experienced some of the weight gain, brain fog, incredible fatigue, feeling as though I was walking through mud, achy joints, digestive problems, and the forgetfulness. My feet would be cold to the bone year round! I was experiencing what Anna had been experiencing for years! I am thankful that I had the background to help myself and knew where to go to get answers. My friends would say, "You don't have hypothyroidism! You're too thin!" If I had not have gone through this with Anna, I would have gained more weight. With what I knew, I knew how to help myself and help my thyroid function better.

Nutrition and fitness have made such a difference in our lives that we formed a health and wellness business, S & A Wellness Duo, and we are making a movement of healing our mission.

CHAPTER 3
The Whole Body Solution

"There are no shortcuts to any place worth going."
– Beverly Sills

Once you have a diagnosis of hypothyroidism and you start taking thyroid hormones, it doesn't stop there. If you stop there, the medication is just a *bandage*. The disease has not been cured. There are some people who start medication and their symptoms go away, and they think all is fine but as time goes on, their symptoms come back and they have to increase their dose. Then, again, as time goes on, their dose increases. Why? They haven't tackled the problem of what has caused them to develop hypothyroidism in the first place and, slowly, the body's immune system is making antibodies that destroy the thyroid. If you do not treat your body's toxic burden, toxins continue to accumulate and impair thyroid function.

Remember we said that researchers now believe over 90 percent of thyroid disease may be autoimmune Hashimoto's thyroiditis. The tests we have currently are not sensitive enough, for many, to pick up the antibodies against the thyroid in the beginning. This was the case with Anna. Her initial diagnosis did not come with complete testing, just the standard TSH test (thyroid stimulating hormone). When we went to the naturopathic doctor in Asheville, they tested her complete thyroid hormone panel and did antibody testing. There were no antibodies in the beginning. The doctor would test for them periodically, and no antibodies were ever found. It took almost 17 years before there were enough antibodies to show up in her lab work.

We were told in the beginning that it was not autoimmune, which at the time, brought some comfort because we know that oftentimes, when you have one autoimmune illness, others may follow. However, this also meant that *all of that time* undetectable antibodies were destroying her thyroid. And yes, her dose increased some through the years. My lab work still shows no antibodies, but with this new research, I will continue to treat my hypothyroidism as if it is autoimmune. Will you be able to get off medication? For some that may be possible, but they still have to do the work to prevent it from coming back. Books that claim to cure disease are misleading because when you have an autoimmune disease, you are never really cured. It may go into remission, but if you continue the lifestyle that caused it in the first place, it will return.

For others, there may be too much damage to completely get off of medication, but it may be possible to reduce the dose. This program will help your thyroid work more efficiently. It will allow your body to make better use of your thyroid hormones. You will feel better! You will lose fat and keep it off! You will stop the progression of disease and stop the onset of other autoimmune issues. This program works for life! Something that you can always come back to and readjust when you get off track. Lifestyle changes are the hardest to make—and ones your doctor will not tell you about or hold your hand—while you make the changes necessary. We will! We're so glad you are here!

In this book, we will teach you what we have learned from our years of getting to the root of the problem, times of getting it right, and times of getting it wrong. It is worth saying again that the suggestions we are giving you are not meant to replace your thyroid medication or to replace your doctor's advice. This should be a complementary approach. Let your doctor know what you are doing and that you are trying to improve your health. You may need to have your thyroid tested more routinely to see if your dose needs reducing. If your doctor isn't cooperative, find a new doctor that will work with you and your goals. We want to help you lose fat and keep it off! We want to help you stop the progression of disease. We want to help you feel your best to be able to get out there and do all of the wonderful things you were meant to do with your life, to live a life full of purpose and not constantly focus on feeling so bad.

Why don't we flip the mindset? Instead of cursing this disorder and settling for this just being the way it is, why don't we embrace it as a warning signal that there is something in our lives that needs changing. If you wallow in self-pity and do nothing about helping yourself, you will surely end up with more chronic diseases in your older years. Most diseases don't happen overnight. They're an accumulation of unhealthful habits over a lifetime. Let's develop healthier habits together.

Our program is a whole-body approach! With any autoimmune issue, it's never about just one aspect of treatment. It's about treating the whole body and the environment in which you surround yourself. We will give you a plan in this book that will give you what you need to get started on the healing pathway.

Mindset. Without the proper mindset, no fat loss program will work. We want to know your goals and your reason for changing your lifestyle to allow healing. What is your motivator?

Then we will talk about the roles of the liver and the digestive system in thyroid function. You will know their role in thyroid hormone conversion and how to cleanse these systems to allow for better function.

We will dive into the causes of leaky gut and how to heal it for better digestive and thyroid function. We will talk about the role the leaky gut plays in causing Hashimoto's disease and other autoimmune issues.

From there we will talk about toxin overload and how to reduce your body's toxic burden. We will give you tools to help your body clean up the waste.

We will talk about sleep and stress and their role in healing. We will give you suggestions for improving sleep and letting go of stress.

We will talk about exercise and the adrenals and adrenal fatigue. We will talk about other hormones important for fat loss. It's not just about the thyroid! Hormones don't work in isolation; they work with other hormones.

We will cover the newest information on genetics and how to prevent those genes involved in hypothyroidism from having an effect. We will cover the new science of Nutrigenomics and biohacking the aging process.

We will talk about overcoming obstacles you may encounter along the way. And at the end we will give you a pathway to take to help you continue to get the results you want and deserve.

Sound like a plan? Let's get to it!

CHAPTER 4

How the Thyroid Functions

*"All illness provides us with an
opportunity to re-evaluate everything."*
— **Cheryl Richardson**

We are going to start out with some startling statistics. Do you know the most prescribed drug in the U.S.? It's Synthroid! This is the synthetic form of thyroid hormone and a T4 only medication. There are 21.5 million prescriptions filled each month for this synthetic thyroid hormone. This is not including the generics, just Synthroid! Crestor, a statin drug to lower cholesterol, is the second most prescribed drug with 21.4 million prescriptions filled each month. What do you hear in TV commercials? Lowering cholesterol! Or about blood pressure or obesity or low libido! You never hear about thyroid disease! Why is it that thyroid disease and thyroid cancer are on the rise? Thyroid cancer has more than doubled since the early 1970s. What has happened over the last two decades that is causing this escalation? It's a question worth asking! According to the American Thyroid Association, 20 million Americans have some form of thyroid disease. One in eight women will develop a thyroid disorder in her lifetime. Undiagnosed or undertreated thyroid disease can lead to more serious conditions like:

- cardiovascular disease;
- infertility;
- mental health issues;
- diabetes;
- obesity;
- heart failure;
- stroke;
- Alzheimer's disease;
- Coma;
- and death.

Pregnant women that are undiagnosed or inadequately treated have an increased risk of miscarriage, preterm delivery, or severe developmental problems in their children. Approximately 80 percent of all thyroid conditions are the autoimmune condition, Hashimoto's thyroiditis. With autoimmune diseases, the body turns on itself and makes antibodies against different parts of the body. In the case of Hashimoto's, the antibodies are made to attack the thyroid quietly and slowly destroy the gland, preventing it from making thyroid hormone. Some researchers say that even though a patient doesn't present with antibodies initially, antibodies could develop later, and the percentage of Hashimoto's might actually be higher. Maybe we should treat all hypothyroid disease as autoimmune Hashimoto's disease. We've seen this first hand.

According to the American Association of Clinical Endocrinologist, thyroid conditions are the number one endocrine disorder in the U.S. We hear about the endocrine disorder, diabetes all day long, but not a single commercial about thyroid disease. There are 20 million people with thyroid disease and 16 million with diabetes. Why are all autoimmune disorders on the rise? What has happened? Is it something in our environment? Is it our diets? Is it our lifestyle? Can we reverse this trend? One thing is for sure—you are not alone.

Let's take just a minute and look at how the thyroid functions in the body so we can become clearer on its importance. It's a little gland located around your larynx on the front of your neck. The thyroid is elegantly called the "Master Gland of Metabolism!" That's because the hormones it makes determine how fast your cells break down food to produce energy. Every cell is dependent on producing enough energy to run all of the processes inside the cell. In high school biology your teacher might have given the analogy that the cell is like a town with little factories called organelles preforming certain functions. All of these organelles need energy to do their job. Every cell has receptor sites on the surface that receive hormones. The hormones instruct the cell to perform a particular task. In the case of thyroid hormone, the active form of the hormone attaches to its receptor and instructs the cell to increase energy production. It directly stimulates the mitochondria, the organelles responsible for producing energy in the form of ATP (adenosine triphosphate), to increase the amount of energy being produced. If the cell can't make enough energy, the cell is weakened and will eventually die.

The thyroid affects every cell and impacts bodily functions like:

- heart rate;
- kidney function;
- skin maintenance;
- growth in children;
- temperature regulation;
- fertility;
- digestion;
- muscle strength;
- water retention;
- hair growth;
- muscle and joint pain;
- activation of the nervous system that leads to higher levels of attention and quicker reflexes, so the lower the function of the thyroid, the lower a person's attention and the slower their reflexes.

So you can see that it controls many functions that are critical for life. Likewise, the symptoms can be so varied and may affect any body system, so your doctor may misdiagnose your condition or maybe not suspect a possible underlying condition of hypothyroidism.

What controls the thyroid gland? The pituitary gland. The pituitary gland is located at the base of the brain and is controlled by the hypothalamus. The hypothalamus monitors the amount of circulating thyroid hormone in the blood and communicates with the pituitary to monitor the hormones of the thyroid. From here, the pituitary assesses the amount of thyroid hormone circulating in the blood and then signals to the thyroid to either speed up or slow down thyroid hormone production. The hormone that the pituitary makes to communicate with the thyroid is called TSH or thyroid stimulating hormone. Conventional doctors used the level of TSH in the blood to determine if the thyroid is functioning properly. The louder the pituitary has to yell at the thyroid to make more hormone (the higher the TSH level will be), the more hypothyroid your body is and the more symptoms you will feel. We will talk about why this isn't a good indicator for thyroid function in a bit.

In order to make the hormones, good nutrients need to be on board. You need iodine, iron, selenium, magnesium, zinc, copper, tyrosine, vitamins E, C and D, and the B vitamins B2, B3, and B6. Vitamins, minerals, and nutrients are so important and their value will be covered more later.

Truth is, conventional medicine doesn't know what causes thyroid disease. There are many variables. If conventional medicine did know of a cause, there would be more drugs developed. No protocol for thyroid disease has been developed since the 1950s when Synthroid was manufactured. Other synthetic forms of T4 have been developed but nothing new about the way hypothyroidism is treated.

Prior to that, doctors used desiccated pig thyroid gland that contained all of the thyroid hormones, not just T4, but there was a problem with standardizing the dose. Each pill could contain a different amount of hormones. That is not the problem today. New technology has allowed manufacturers to standardize desiccated thyroid hormone with precise dosing. For many, desiccated thyroid hormone gives better results because it contains all of the hormones produced by the thyroid and is a natural product, not synthetic, so the body has an easier time using the hormones. Some people get better results on a compounded T4/T3 medication. Work with your doctor to decide which approach is better for you. Make sure to work with a doctor that knows how to properly dose desiccated thyroid hormones if you want to try this natural product.

Anna and I have both used synthetic, desiccated, and compounded medication through the years. Personally, when I was on synthetic Synthroid and Levoxyl, my joints hurt so badly that I couldn't workout and the pain kept me from sleeping. I do better on desiccated thyroid. I have been able to lower my dose since the beginning of my thyroid disease and have been stabilized for years. Anna is currently on a compounded T4/T3 medication and doing well on that.

Research came out in 2012 from the National Academy of Hypothyroidism looking at our current ways of testing for the presence or absence of thyroid disease by using only TSH levels. The research showed that TSH testing alone does not give the whole picture of thyroid health. Naturopathic medicine had known this for some time and had been using other tests to indicate the presence of disease. We will post the tests used by our doctors on our website that give a more complete picture of thyroid health. We will summarize these results of that research. Please excuse all of the science here, but it's important to talk about this to explain why you are still having hypothyroid symptoms.

THYROID HORMONES

There are several hormones that we know the thyroid produces: T0, T1, T2, T3, T4, and Calcitonin. The number indicates the number of iodine atoms that are attached to the hormone. We don't know the function of T0, T1, and T2, but there is some indication that T2 works in helping with fat loss and being able to maintain the fat loss. It is also thought to help with muscle gain and preventing insulin resistance and works in conjunction with T3. More research is needed. Calcitonin increases bone calcium content and helps to regulate calcium and phosphorus levels in the blood.

We are going to talk mainly about the major hormones, T4 (Thyroxine) and T3 (Triiodothyronine). The thyroid makes mainly T4, which is the inactive form of thyroid hormone. It has to be converted to the active form T3 in order to fit onto the receptors of the cell to influence energy production and speed up metabolism. Synthetic forms of thyroid hormone are T4 only preparation and depend on the body's ability to convert it to the active form, T3. Desiccated thyroid hormone contain all of the thyroid hormones but only the T4 and T3 are standardized.

Thyroxine, T4, is needed to convert riboflavin, vitamin B2, to FAD (flavin adenine dinucleotide), a molecule necessary for cellular respiration and energy production in the cell. If someone is on T3 only medication, they may not be making enough FAD for energy production and might experience fatigue.

The conversion of T4 to the active form, T3, takes place in various parts of the body. The liver is the major player with 60 percent of the conversion taking place here! A healthy liver is vital for a healthy thyroid. Twenty percent of the conversion happens in the intestines and 20 percent happens in other tissues like the muscles. We will be discussing ways to clean up the liver and intestines to make conversion of thyroid hormone more effective. Oftentimes, it's not about the amount of hormone you are making or taking but about the ability to convert it into a useable form. This can also be why your thyroid tests come back normal, but you still have hypothyroid symptoms.

ENZYMES NECESSARY FOR THE CONVERSION OF T4 TO T3

Deiodinase enzymes are responsible for activation or deactivation of thyroid hormones in the body. There are three that we know about: D1, D2, and D3 (Deiodinase 1, 2 and 3).

D1 is found in the body tissues, like the muscles, and converts T4 into the active form T3. This enzyme is *not* found in the pituitary.

D2 if found mainly in the pituitary and not in body tissues and is 1000 times better at converting T4 into T3 than D1.

D3 is only found in the tissues and *not* the pituitary, and converts T4 into RT3 (reverse T3), which is an inactive form of hormone and clogs the receptor sites on the surface of the cell so that T3 can't attach. Consequently, metabolism slows down because it interferes with energy production.

In the naturopathic world, TSH has not been used as the only indicator of thyroid function for some time, because it does not indicate the level of active T3 in the body tissues. The pituitary is under a completely different enzyme system and the amount of active T3 will always be higher in the pituitary than the rest of the body. When someone has even a slightly elevated TSH (higher in the normal range), the amount of T3 in the tissues of the body can be deficient and hypothyroid symptoms will be present, but their bloodwork will be in the *normal range*. When the TSH gets high enough to be *out of range*, a person will be struggling with severe hypothyroidism.

In addition, this study found that tissue levels of T3 drop dramatically out of proportion to serum T3 levels. Serum T3 may drop by 30 percent, but tissue T3 levels may drop by a greater degree, 70-80 percent. So your bloodwork may come back in the normal range, but your tissue is still deficient and you are still experiencing symptoms. The level of T3 in the tissues is important for being able to affect the cell and increase metabolism.

Remember that the pituitary doesn't have D3. It competes with D1 to convert T4 into RT3 (inactive form that clogs the receptors), thereby preventing T3 from attaching, reducing metabolism. Even small increases in RT3 can cause significant increase in hypothyroid symptoms. If your doctor adds more T4 only medication, like Synthroid, more RT3 can be made.

CLASSIC SYMPTOMS OF HYPOTHYROIDISM

Symptoms for hypothyroidism might include: weight gain, fatigue, hair loss, sensitivity to cold, constipation, dry skin, puffiness, high cholesterol, sluggishness, foggy brain, memory problems, infertility, carpal tunnel syndrome, swelling of the thyroid, changes in menstrual cycle, and fertility problems.

CAUSES OF HYPOTHYROIDISM

Research conducted by the National Academy of Hypothyroidism looked at why the conventional test for thyroid function, the TSH test, was a poor indicator of thyroid function. Here is a summary of some of the causes of hypothyroidism that they found related to a poor thyroid hormone conversion.

CHRONIC STRESS

Whether stress is physical, mental, or chemical, chronic stress suppresses D1 activity in the tissues and increases D3 so more RT3 is made. This leads to hypothyroid symptoms like weight gain, fatigue, depression. Chronic stress raises cortisol and suppresses immunity. When stress is treated with prednisone or other glucocorticoids, D1 activity is decreased and D3 is increased adding to hypothyroid symptoms of decrease in metabolism and energy production and weight gain. We will show you ways we reduce stress later in the book.

DEPRESSION

Many people who suffer from depression have an underlying undiagnosed thyroid condition. Like with chronic stress, depression causes a decrease in D1 activity and a decrease in the ability to get T4 into the cells, resulting in lower intracellular levels of T4. Other research shows that there is a defective transport protein that carries T4 across the brain barrier so there is less hormone in the brain. If you or someone you know suffers from depression, tell them to have a complete thyroid panel run by their doctor.

CHRONIC PAIN

Chronic pain suppresses D1 in the tissues but it upregulates the activity of D2 in the pituitary, so no signal is sent to the thyroid to increase T4 production. The tissues will be deficient in T3 and the person will experience hypothyroid symptoms. Pain medications can help to alleviate the pain, but they also decrease D1 activity.

ACUTE OR CHRONIC DIETING

Calorie restriction can significantly reduce the amount of T3 circulating in the blood and inside the cell by 50 percent! It does this by causing a decrease in D1 activity. That significantly reduces metabolism and often takes years to restore to normal. The body stays in starvation mode despite returning to a normal food intake. In addition, D2 in the pituitary was shown to increase activity resulting in no change in the TSH activity. This means that the hypothyroid symptoms will be experienced but will not show up on a TSH test. This makes it very difficult to lose and to maintain weight. This flies in the face of the "eat less and exercise more" mentality.

Other research shows that people who have gained weight in the past and have lost weight by calorie restriction had significantly lower metabolisms (25 percent lower) than those who weigh the same but had not gained or lost significant weight in the past. This equates to a deficit of 500-600 calories a day or jogging 1.5 hours a day just to maintain weight loss.

This is a great example of those people on reality weight loss shows that lose tremendous amounts of weight on the show, but when they get back to their real lives, the weight plus more comes back quickly.

There is a way to repair a damaged metabolism, and our program will help put you on the road to recovery.

INSULIN RESISTANCE/DIABETES/ METABOLIC SYNDROME/OBESITY

All of these disorders have significant reduction in conversion of T4 to T3 and an increase in RT3 by reducing D1 activity and increasing D3. And again, D2 is upregulated so the TSH will be unchanged or decreased, making it an unreliable indicator of thyroid function.

LEPTIN RESISTANCE

Leptin is a hormone secreted by the fat tissue that tells the hypothalamus (part of the brain) that there is enough fat in the body and to slow down hunger and to increase metabolism to increase burning of the extra fat (lipolysis). It opposes the action of ghrelin, the hunger hormone, secreted by the gastrointestinal track. We will talk more about these two hormones later.

Leptin resistance comes from chronically overeating and the brain doesn't hear leptin signaling to slow down hunger. The action of D1 is decreased and D3 is increased, resulting in more RT3 lowering metabolism. Again, pituitary D2 is upregulated so there is no change or a suppression of TSH, making it an unreliable indicator of thyroid problems.

EXERCISE

People who perform long duration, moderate intensity exercise like running long distances, and who combine this with dieting, lower D1 activity and increase D3.

IRON DEFICIENCY

Iron deficiency has been shown to significantly reduce T4 to T3 conversion and increase D3 activity, lowering metabolism with unchanged TSH.

INFLAMMATION

Inflammation is the root cause of many diseases. Inflammatory cytokines like IL-1, IL-6 (Interleukin-1, Interleukin-6), CRP (C-Reactive Protein), and TNF-alpha (Tumor Necrosis factor—alpha), will significantly reduce D1 activity and decrease T3 levels. Inflammatory conditions would include stress, obesity, diabetes, depression, menopause, heart disease, autoimmune conditions (lupus, Hashimoto's, MS, arthritis, etc.), injury, chronic infections, and cancer. All of these conditions lead to a decreased T4 to T3 conversion in the body tissues and the experience of hypothyroid symptoms. We will show you how to significantly reduce inflammation to improve T4 to T3 conversion.

ENVIRONMENTAL TOXINS

Many toxins like plastics (BPA but there are others), pesticides, mercury and other heavy metals, and flame retardants like PBDE and others, are known to suppress thyroid function by physically blocking thyroid receptors and reducing T4 to T3 conversion. Small amounts of toxins are all that is required to have a profound effect on energy production and metabolism. We will explore more about toxins later in the book.

LOW TESTOSTERONE

Low testosterone in men and in women will lower D1 activity, again, without changing the TSH levels. We will talk about natural ways to increase testosterone levels to improve conversion.

HUMAN GROWTH HORMONE

A deficiency in human growth hormone will reduce D1 activity and increase D3 without changing TSH levels. We will discuss ways to raise your HGH naturally to improve hormone conversion.

In summary, there are many causes of thyroid disease. In addition to the ones researched by NAH, there are other causes that would include: having a genetic predisposition, chronic infections including Epstein Barr and Lyme disease, food allergies and sensitivities, leaky gut/gut dysbiosis, hormone imbalances,

Factors That Affect Thyroid Function

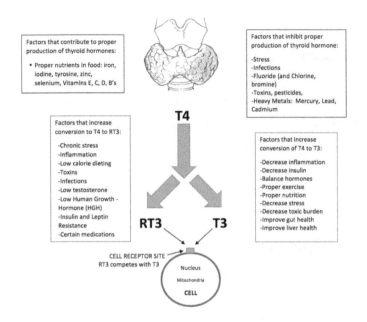

Factors that contribute to proper production of thyroid hormones:

- Proper nutrients in food: iron, iodine, tyrosine, zinc, selenium, Vitamins E, C, D, B's

Factors that inhibit proper production of thyroid hormone:

-Stress
-Infections
-Fluoride (and Chlorine, bromine)
-Toxins, pesticides,
-Heavy Metals: Mercury, Lead, Cadmium

Factors that increase conversion to T4 to RT3:

-Chronic stress
-Inflammation
-Low calorie dieting
-Toxins
-Infections
-Low testosterone
-Low Human Growth - Hormone (HGH)
-Insulin and Leptin Resistance
-Certain medications

Factors that increase conversion of T4 to T3:

-Decrease inflammation
-Decrease insulin
-Balance hormones
-Proper exercise
-Proper nutrition
-Decrease stress
-Decrease toxic burden
-Improve gut health
-Improve liver health

T4

RT3   **T3**

CELL RECEPTOR SITE
RT3 competes with T3

Nucleus

Mitochondria

CELL

insulin and leptin resistance, nutritional deficiencies, inactivity, and adrenal fatigue.

From all of this research, it is abundantly clear that the cause of hypothyroidism can have many triggers. It is more than just taking thyroid hormone that is needed. It is a whole body approach.

In the following chapters, we will address lifestyle changes that will help to improve thyroid health. We will help you achieve better thyroid hormone conversion to improve metabolism. Improving thyroid health and improving thyroid hormone conversion will boost your energy level to help you take back your life!

Let's get to it!

CHAPTER 5
Get Your Brain Onboard

"The mind is the most important part of achieving any fitness goal. Mental change always comes before physical change."

– Matt McGorry

With hypothyroidism, there can be some level of "melancholy", or feelings of being stuck with no way out. In some it can be more like depression, which can make wanting to change, the motivation to change, and the drive to change that much harder. Remember that when you are stressed or depressed, less active thyroid hormone (T3) is made in your tissues leading to more hypothyroid symptoms. We have to pull ourselves up out of this slump which all starts with your mind. Here are some things we have found to be helpful in focusing on moving forward instead of staying in that place of despair.

Before any real change in lifestyle or diet can occur, you have to deal with your mind. Our minds can often be self-sabotaging with lots of negative talk and negative energy that keeps us from moving ahead. Staying where you are is the easiest thing to do. Change requires effort. There is no instant reward. No quick fix and so this is where most of us stop and simply give up. In order to really change, you have to dig deep and put that negative self-talk behind you and move forward. We are going to cover three areas of changing your mind that we feel are important to allow true change to occur and stick. Come back to these things if you feel yourself slipping backward. Let's talk about *motivation*, *mindset*, and *mindfulness*.

MOTIVATION

What motivates you to want to change and to lose weight and feel better? Is it perhaps wanting to look great at the beach, or looking good for your husband. Let's dig deeper than that. What about changing to improve your health, or to have more energy for your children and to be a role model for them, or changing to be able to live longer to one day be able to play with your grandchildren? Sometimes, something happens that causes us to make the decision that now is the time. This is called your *why*. Whatever this is for you, write it down and post it where you will see it every morning. It is crucial that your *why* be bigger, stronger and worth more than any excuse you have to stay where you are. This is what will keep you pushing forward no matter how bad those days can be. Here are some steps to help you get motivated for change.

1. Find your *why*.

    Post your *why* on your mirror in your bathroom or tuck it into a space where you will see it first thing every morning. Read it every morning. Some say your *why* has to make you cry. Not so sure about that, but it does need to evoke a feeling that is stronger than your willingness to settle for the status quo. Let's make a vision board. We have found this to be really helpful in clarifying specific life goals. These boards reinforce your daily intentions and affirmations. Cut out pictures and quotes from magazines that would represent your hopes and dreams of what your future would look like when your dreams are accomplished. Paste these on a poster board and put it where you can see it daily. This is something that you can look at and retrain your brain to look at your future as if it were now. You are learning to look forward instead of looking at the present or even the past.

2. Write down your goals.

    What are your long-term goals, where do you want to be in six months to a year? Then, determine your weekly and daily goals to help you accomplish your long-term goals. Studies show that when you write down your goals you are more likely to achieve them. Most of us go through life as if the script has already been written and we are powerless to change our situation. We do have the power! It takes a plan! All successful people have plans to help them accomplish their desires—whether it is in business or a body change, a plan is a must. Nothing happens haphazardly.

3. Find a support group.

When you are trying to change, it can often be a challenge if you are not getting support from family or friends or a spouse. In these cases you must look at your *why* to remember the reason you are wanting to change. Try to find a gym, a workout buddy who has the same goals, or meet up groups to go walking, to act as accountability partners for you. It can be discouraging when you feel like you are the only one wanting to change. That being said, not having a support group is not an excuse to not do the work. Always remember, you are doing this for you!

4. Approve of yourself just the way you are today.

You've heard the old saying, "If it's meant to be, it's up to me," well the same holds true with self-love. You must love yourself today, as the beautiful person you are, and for the trials and tribulations that got you where you are *today*. Negative self-talk takes you down that rabbit hole that leads to pity and shame and it makes it hard to resurface. It will not motivate you to do the things you need to do to make the changes you want. This is a journey and not a sprint. These changes are meant to be for a lifetime. Another favorite quote of ours is by Henry Ford, "Whether you think you can, or think you can't—you are right." This quote is so powerful, right? Change, motivation, drive, and focus all start and end in the mind. Every single person on this planet is unique; with no two stories the same. This is your journey; not the next person or the next. Your journey and your story is what set you apart, so embrace yourself for where you are right now.

5. Say positive daily affirmations.

Saying positive daily affirmations about yourself builds your mental toughness. Create a morning mantra and recite it every morning along with reading your *why*. Recite your mantra several times a day and especially when you are in a tough situation. It will help you get through it. Say things like: *I am worthy of self-care, I will make healthy choices today. I will work out because I love my body. I am feeling healthier and stronger each day. I am learning how to love my body. Everything I eat heals me and nourishes me. I am deserving.* Google positive affirmations if you need help coming up with some that fit your situation.

6. Establish a reward system.

When you have had a really good week of meeting your goals, set up a reward system for yourself. Go and get a pedicure, or a massage, or buy yourself a pair of shoes. Whatever it is, you deserve to reward yourself for all of your great effort.

7. Stop making excuses.

So many people say that they will wait for the New Year to get started, or they will wait until Monday or after their vacation or maybe when they can afford a gym membership, or maybe they think they just don't have the time. All of these things are just ways to procrastinate. There is no time like the present. Excuses are an easy way out. Stop hiding all of your potential behind a long list of good-for-nothing excuses. You can either have major positive life change, or your bag of excuses, not both, so make a decision to go for it. This is the reason your *why* needs to truly reflect where you want to go.

8. Don't let perfection be the enemy of progress.

    Do your best every day to reach your daily goals. Don't beat yourself up if you backslide. Just acknowledge the fact and get back on track then. Don't say, *Well, I've blown it so I might as well blow the whole weekend!* Get right back on track with the next meal or the next workout.

    Just like one healthy meal isn't going to change your health status, one bad meal or one missed workout isn't going to derail your entire efforts. Just get back up and get back on that horse.

9. Develop a routine that becomes second nature.

    With practice, your new diet and lifestyle will become effortless. You will know what works and what doesn't. Your food choices will come automatically. Your workouts will be scheduled. It's like being on autopilot.

10. Journal.

    It is really important to journal your feelings, your mantra, keeping track of food, water intake, and workouts. More about this later.

MINDSET SHIFTS

Changing your diet and lifestyle requires a shift in your mindset. Don't come into this from a negative mindset, focusing on all of your trouble spots like, *I have such a big belly*, or *I hate the way my muffin top rolls over my waistband*, or *My arms are so flabby I never go sleeveless*. Focusing on your trouble spots makes you obsess about having to *fix* yourself. Instead, focus on your *why* and think about all of the good things that will come with losing weight like—better health, more energy to enjoy your family, and living healthier as you age. Studies show that the more dissatisfied women are with the way their bodies look, the more likely they will not make the changes necessary to lose weight and get healthy. Simply thinking that you are overweight is self-fulfilling and actually leads to more weight gain. How you see yourself predicts your actions. Let's change our mindsets!

1. Express Gratitude and Positivity

    It is hard to make healthy choices when you feel stressed or frustrated. It's hard to put together a nice salad or go get your workout in when you are anxious or upset. At times when you are not stressed, the same tasks are effortless. It's hard to stick to your fitness goals when you are stressed out about balancing family obligations with work and your own personal needs. It may feel selfish. Remember that you are no good to anyone when you are sick. Showing *gratitude* is one way to stay *positive* and helps put things in perspective. It helps you see what's really important. Studies have actually shown that programs that used methods that encourage positive beliefs in the participant's ability to reach their weight loss goals have improved eating habits that allow their goals to be met. Gratitude is a powerful tool. Start a *Gratitude Journal*. Each day, write down five things that you are grateful for each day. So it becomes a habit to remember to be grateful, set your alarm on your phone or computer several times a day, and when it goes off, take five minutes to take a breath and write down five things that you are grateful for—and acknowledge those things. This deliberate practice throughout the day will strengthen your mental toughness and will lower stress and help you feel more grounded.

2.   Identify Your *Trouble Thoughts*.

When negative self-talk enters your mind, turn that thought around. Say to yourself to stop the thought. Say your mantra to yourself. Write the negative thought in your journal, and try to determine why the thought came up to begin with and what you did to turn that thought around. By writing it in your journal, you can see if there is a pattern to your thoughts and what brings them up for you.

MINDFULNESS

So many of us are guilty for going through our day without being mindful about what we are eating, how much we are eating, or knowing if we ate a vegetable that day. We are unaware of how much we sit during the day. The practice of mindfulness actually comes from the Buddhist Monks. They are very aware of what is happening within their bodies and in their surroundings. We can use this practice to help reduce our stress and to become more in touch with ourselves. Mindfulness is important in weight loss. When eating, slow down. Notice the color of the food, the way it smells, the flavors in the food, its texture. Chew your food slowly and completely. Get rid of any distractions like your cell phone, the television, or reading while you are eating. Notice how the food makes you feel.

The Gut Mind Connection. Have you ever been upset with someone and eaten a meal? Maybe you're upset with a coworker or your spouse and you are talking about that over lunch with your friend. After the meal, you have an upset stomach and feel bloated, or maybe feel something like indigestion. Digestion is a complex process requiring energy and hormonal signals that occur between the gut and the brain (more on this later). These signals tell the brain that you are full and to stop eating. It takes about 20 minutes for the brain to register this signal. When you eat too quickly, you can overeat before the brain has time to register the signal of being full. When you overeat, there may not be enough enzymes produced to digest all of the food that has been eaten. When you eat when you are upset, enzymes might not be fully released and in both instances, we feel stomach upsets and bloating. Here are some pointers to be more mindful when eating.

1. Stop before you eat that snack.
   Understand why you are eating. Are you hungry because you skipped breakfast or lunch? Are you thirsty? Oftentimes, feelings of hunger are actually

signs of dehydration, so drink a glass of water before you eat. Are you bored, or upset, or worried? Being aware of why you are eating helps you understand your relationship with food. So many times we scarf something down so quickly, and immediately we regret our food choice because we didn't think before we ate. If this happens, acknowledge this, and move on. Make pre-planning a priority.

2. Say grace before you eat, or acknowledge that the food you are eating is for your body's nourishment.
   This practice slows you down and makes you more mindful of what you are eating.

3. Chew your food thoroughly before swallowing it.
   Digestion begins in the mouth. Food should be chewed thoroughly before swallowing to allow it to mix with salivary juices to begin the digestive process. Practice chewing each mouthful 30 times before swallowing. This will slow you down and allow your digestive system to be able to absorb more of the nutrients in the food.

4. Drink a large glass of water 30 minutes before you eat.
   This will prepare the digestive system for food and will help you not eat as much because you will be less hungry. Do not drink much at all during the meal to allow the enzymes to stay concentrated for better digestion.

5. Eat a vibrant, colorful plate of food.
   The more color on your plate, the more nutrients you will be consuming.

6. Wait before getting seconds.
    Give your brain time to send the signal of being full.

Motivation, mindset and mindfulness are powerful tools to rewire the brain. This is so important with any type of change you are getting ready to embark upon.

So in summary, remember your *why*. Write down your goals. Make a vision board for clarity. Find a support group. Get rid of negative self-talk. Use daily affirmations to begin to think more positively about yourself. Give yourself rewards when you've accomplished a goal. Journal your thoughts. Express gratitude for the wonderful things in your life. Be mindful of what you are eating and doing. Awareness is the key to being able to change bad habits!

CHAPTER 6

Leaky Gut. Is it a Thing?

*"To keep the body in good health is a duty ... otherwise
we shall not be able to keep our mind strong and clear."*
– Buddha

Our gut is one of the most important metabolic organs
in our body. It has the responsibility of digesting this
foreign material called food, into small molecules that
are recognizable by the body so our immune systems don't
react when we absorb the nutrients. How remarkable is that?
The gut is also the second most concentrated area of nerve
tissue in the body outside of the brain and spinal cord. It
is often called our second brain. Almost two thirds of our
immune cells and many of our neurotransmitters are produced
here as well. Remember too, that this is the site of 20 percent

of thyroid hormone conversion, T4 to T3. Keeping it healthy is paramount.

The gut is lined with mucus secreting cells that lay down a protective mucus barrier. Underneath the mucus are the enterocytes, the cells that make up the interior intestinal wall. They are lined with microvilli on the surface of the cell pointing towards the inside of the intestinal track. The microvilli allow a greater surface area for nutrients to pass through into the enterocyte and then into the capillaries that lie beneath them. The enterocytes are held together by tight junctions that act like rivets attaching one cell to the next. This prevents passage of larger, undigested food particles and pathogens into the bloodstream. If the gut becomes inflamed it causes these tight junctions to disconnect making a gap in the wall that allows larger, undigested molecules to get through and into the bloodstream. The immune system sees these larger molecules as foreign and mounts an immune attack producing antibodies against the invader. These antibodies get confused and start attacking proteins in the body that have a similar molecular structure. This is called *molecular mimicry*. In the case of Hashimoto's, these antibodies attack the thyroid. In arthritis, the antibodies attack the joint tissue. In diabetes, they attack the pancreas, etc.

If you ask your conventional doctor if there is a disease condition called leaky gut, they will probably say no. The conventional medical community does not recognize leaky gut as a condition because there is no drug or protocol to treat it. It is healed through eliminating triggers. Therefore, doctors don't recognize it as real, only hype from the naturopathic medical community.

We said earlier that 90 percent of all thyroid disorders could be Hashimoto's. The antibodies produced against the thyroid are slowly destroying the tissue and therefore, the amount of thyroid hormones that it can make decreases. Once you've been diagnosed with Hashimoto's, other autoimmune disorders can develop. Taking thyroid replacement hormones can slow the progression to some degree but unless the underlying trigger is determined and stopped, the destruction of the thyroid slowly continues.

Autoimmune disorders are never cured. We can, however, put them into remission, which is the good news here. In order for Hashimoto's disease, and other autoimmune disorders, to occur, several things must be in place: a genetic predisposition, triggers that cause the genes to be expressed, and intestinal permeability or leaky gut. If we can stop the triggers and heal leaky gut, the genes will no longer be expressed and Hashimoto's will be in remission. You will no longer have hypothyroid symptoms and you will be able to lose the weight and keep it off and be filled with energy!

PREVENTING LEAKY GUT

Even though we can't do anything about the genes we inherit, we can prevent them from having an effect and becoming expressed. One of those ways is to find your personal triggers that cause leaky gut and get rid of those triggers so leaky gut can be healed. What are some of those triggers?

SUGAR, HIGH FRUCTOSE CORN SYRUP, AND NATURAL SWEETENERS

When I was doing my research when Anna was first diagnosed with hypothyroidism, I came across one doctor that recommended his patients with hypothyroidism follow the same diet he gave to his diabetic patients; one low in sugar and starchy carbohydrates. This was the only recommendation I could find at that time. We immediately cut out the sugar! No more sodas, no more sweet tea, no more fruit juices. We learned how to drink water!

Since this time, it has been found that sugar is the driving force behind many diseases such as diabetes, heart disease, obesity, cancer and so many more. Sugar is the biggest culprit in high cholesterol and has been found to be as addictive as cocaine! In 2012, a 60 Minutes Documentary, entitled *Is Sugar Toxic?* aired. Scientists from the University of California discovered that when sugar is consumed, the fructose in sugar is converted to the small dense LDL cholesterol particles that are so dangerous in causing heart disease. This was the beginning of the discovery that excess sugar in the diet, more so than fat, is the cause of cholesterol problems. As a result, the scientists recommended that men get no more than 37 grams of sugar a day and women get no more than 25 grams a day. To put that in prospective, a single coke has 39 grams of sugar. Keep track of the sugar you are consuming and you will probably be shocked.

Sugar causes the overgrowth of the yeast Candida, and bad bacteria in the gut that leads to inflammation and leaky gut. Candida causes you to crave even more sugar because that is what it feeds on. The more sugar you eat, the more Candida—and the more you crave sugar. It's a vicious cycle. Some researchers think that Candida is the root cause of leaky gut and autoimmunity. Candida produce little roots called hyphae and they bore through the intestinal wall producing little holes that allow those larger undigested particles to get into the bloodstream and cause the autoimmune response. Candida can also leak out and get into the bloodstream causing systemic Candida. This can cause fatigue, depression, anxiety, skin eruptions, immune system malfunctions, brain fog, joint aches, and feeling drunk or dizzy! A waste product of Candida is acetaldehyde which is a byproduct of alcohol metabolism which contributes to that drunk feeling.

High fructose corn syrup might be more dangerous than sugar. Sugar is 50 percent glucose and 50 percent fructose. High fructose corn syrup is processed so that the fructose is concentrated and makes up more of the syrup, anywhere from 55 percent to 75 percent fructose. The problem with fructose is that it is not used as an energy source, like glucose, and has to be broken down by the liver, thereby consuming energy in the process. The liver converts fructose to fat and stores it in the belly and in the liver itself. Glucose is transported to the cells where it can be used to make energy. Over-consumption of fructose scars the liver leading to fatty liver disease, driving obesity, diabetes, cancer, and heart disease. Along with sugar, fructose causes leaky gut.

Read your labels! High fructose corn syrup is used to sweeten many processed foods, sodas, and candies. It is cheaper than sugar so the industry chooses this over sugar. Fructose is found in small amounts in fruits and does not seem to cause the same problems as fructose sweeteners. Choose less sweet fruits like berries to decrease the amount of sugar you are eating. Be careful of the hybrid fruits available today because they are bred to be sweeter than normal. Do not drink fruit juices as they contain more fructose. If you like green juices, be careful of the amount of fruit that they contain. The more fruit, the more sugar. Go for less fruit in your juices. Our juice cleanse is filled with low sugar juice options that are delicious and powerfully cleansing to the body.

So where do all of the other sweeteners fit into the picture? Whether it is coconut sugar, agave, maple syrup, honey, it doesn't matter! Sugar is sugar. They all cause leaky gut, a surge in insulin, add to fat gain, especially around the waist, as well as weight gain. The amount of sugar must be drastically reduced in order to lose weight, help the thyroid function better, heal leaky gut, and reduce the progress of Hashimoto's.

Don't think this gives the green light for artificial sweeteners! They can be just as damaging to the body. They are synthetic so the liver has to break them down, and they can add to the toxicity of the liver. Remember the liver is where 60 percent of thyroid hormone conversion takes place, T4 to T3! If it is spending time breaking down synthetics, then it has less time to convert precious thyroid hormone. Studies have shown that people who use artificial sweeteners are less sensitive to sweet taste, and so it takes more sweetener to satisfy them. In addition, people who use artificial sweeteners or who drink diet drinks will eat larger portions of sweets, like cake or dessert, than people who do not use artificial sweeteners. Studies also indicate that just the taste of sweetness causes a surge in insulin production and promotes fat storage. In order to lose weight insulin must be controlled. More on this later.

Action steps: Drink lots of clean, filtered water, (half your body weight in ounces per day as a general rule). Squeeze the juice from a wedge of lemon or orange into your water to make it more palatable if needed. Use slices of cucumbers and mint leaves in your water. Eat a piece of fruit for that sugar fix instead of a candy bar. Try having just one or two bites of a dessert instead of a whole serving. If you are addicted to sugar, try cutting the amount you use in half for a couple of days, then cut that amount in half and so on, until you have cut it out of your diet.

ELIMINATE GLUTEN AND PROCESSED GRAINS

Gluten is a large, sticky protein found in grains like wheat, barley, and rye. This protein is very hard to digest and undigested fragments of gluten cause the enterocytes to release a protein called zonulin. Zonulin is responsible for controlling gut permeability and when it is present in high amounts, as triggered by the undigested gluten particle, the gut becomes more inflamed and more permeable. The tight junctions break open and the larger undigested gluten molecules pass into the bloodstream causing an immune response. This was thought to only be a problem with Celiac disease, but now, researchers are finding that even if you don't have the genes for Celiac, other genes may be present that cause gluten to be a problem by causing a rise in zonulin. It is estimated that 50 percent or more of the people suffer from gluten intolerance. Gluten exhibits molecular mimicry with the thyroid meaning gluten's molecular structure is similar to the thyroid and the antibodies produced will attack the thyroid tissue resulting in Hashimoto's.

Bread, whether white, whole-wheat, or gluten free, is made by grinding the grains into small particle sizes that causes it to be digested very quickly and will send insulin skyrocketing. It is a processed starch. Starch is nothing more than glucose molecules strung together, and when digested, lots of glucose is produced. This leads to fat storage. Insulin must be controlled in order to lose weight. Get your fiber from vegetables, nuts, and seeds like flax and chia seeds.

Action steps: Avoid wheat and all wheat products. Avoid other gluten containing grains. Avoid gluten-free processed foods because they tend to cause just as large of an insulin surge as wheat, which causes fat storage. Use lettuce or collards to make a wrap instead of using bread. Eat salads. Read labels! Beer is made from barley which is a gluten containing grain and should be avoided. If you do use gluten-free products, watch the portion size and only use these occasionally.

AVOID DAIRY

Like gluten, dairy is one of the top foods that causes allergic reactions. Dairy contains two proteins, casein and whey, that can be problematic. Just like gluten, these proteins are hard to digest and can cause inflammation in the gut that leads to leaky gut increasing the chance of autoimmunity. Like gluten, dairy proteins have a similar molecular structure as the thyroid tissue and exhibit molecular mimicry. The antibodies made against the undigested casein and whey proteins leak out of the gut and mount an immune response making antibodies that will attack the thyroid.

Dairy leads to fat gain due to the high amounts of the sugar lactose. Even though it scores low on the glycemic index, it is the combination of fat and sugar that leads to weight gain. It is a hefty source of calories per ounce and can easily be overeaten. Cheese was one of the hardest things to give up for us! It's probably the same for you. The reason for this is that the protein casein is very addictive. Nature made it so! It causes the calf to want to come back to its mother to feed. It's the perfect food for baby cows! In cheese, the casein is concentrated, making it that much more addictive!

You ask where you will get your calcium. There is calcium in nuts, seeds, and greens. Contrary to popular belief, dairy has been found to be bad for your bones. It tends to increase the acidity of the body and leaches calcium from the bones—and may actually contribute to osteoporosis.

Action Steps: Use almond milk or coconut milk or another nut milk as a dairy substitute. Avoid soy because it contains isoflavones that may adversely affect the thyroid. We like to grind up pine nuts and sprinkle them on a salad. It tastes a little like parmesan cheese. Use nutritional yeast to give you a cheesy taste. Its good sprinkled on popcorn. Use a pea protein powder or a hemp protein powder instead of whey.

AVOID FATS THAT ARE INFLAMMATORY

There has been a drastic change in the ratio of omega-6 and omega-3 consumed in the American diet over the last 50 years that has contributed to the epidemic of modern diseases.

Omega-6 fats come mainly from seeds like safflower, sunflower, corn, cottonseed, sesame, canola, and peanut oils. Omega-3 oils fats come from fish, flaxseed, chia seed, and walnuts and are so important in brain health and heart health and overall health in general. We need both types, but the problem comes from getting too many omega-6 fats in our diet and not enough omega-3 fats. It has been estimated that our ancestors ate a diet that was closer to half omega 6 fats and half omega 3 fats. In the 1930s, we ate twice as much omega-6 fats as omega-3 fats. And today we are eating 1,000 times more omega-6 than omega-3 fats! Americans get almost 20 percent of their calories from soybean oil!

Where are they getting so much omega-6 in their diets? Fast foods and processed foods! This is so inflammatory to the gut and throughout the body! You are the fat that you eat! The fat that you eat makes up the fat in the cell membranes and changes how fluid the membranes are and how hormones communicate with the receptors on the surface. Too much omega-6 (polyunsaturated) makes the cell membrane too fluid. Too much saturated fats makes the membrane too rigid. You need the right combination of fats in the cell membrane to make it have just the right amount of flexibility. Hormones can't attach well and materials can get in and out too easily when it's too fluid. When it's too stiff, hormone receptors decline in number and make it harder for hormones to find a receptor and attach. We want the goldilocks' effect; just right!

Action steps: So how do we correct the ratio? Stop eating fast food! Stop eating processed foods! They are loaded in omega-6 fats! Eating fatty fish like wild-caught salmon and not farm- raised. Farm-raised fish have more omega-6 oils that will not improve your ratio. Eat organic, grass-fed, pasture-raised meats and eggs for the same reason. Conventionally raised meats have more omega-6 fats. Use extra virgin, cold pressed olive oil (make sure it is real olive oil and not adulterated with cheaper fats) and organic coconut oil, and ditch the canola oil. Eat fats in their natural form like avocados, olives, or a palm full of nuts or seeds. Take a high-quality fish oil supplement. Fish oil supplements should not smell too fishy or cause you to burp up fishy tastes in the back of the throat. That is an indication of oil that is rancid. Make sure your oil is free of heavy metals like mercury as toxins are stored in the fat tissue. Any animal fat you consume needs to be organic and grass-fed.

OTHER TRIGGERS

Other triggers for leaky gut are some prescription drugs like antibiotics and over the counter drugs like NSAIDS, food allergies or food sensitivities, too much alcohol, strenuous exercise, Crohn's disease, ulcerative colitis, celiac disease to name a few.

Trying to figure out the best diet can be a confusing task. There are so many experts telling you to eat this diet or you will lose weight on this one or lose weight drinking this coffee. Eat paleo. Eat keto. Eat vegan. Try intermittent fasting! Instead of grabbing on to the latest fad diet, let's figure out the right diet for you. It will be one that improves your bloodwork. One that improves your symptoms. One that allows you to heal and lose weight. It's one that you can do for a lifetime. So many diets out there are just not sustainable. You may lose some weight but regain it when you can no longer stick to it. Let's figure out the best one for you!

SO, WHAT'S THE TAKEAWAY?

The first things that must happen to heal Hashimoto's disease is to reduce the inflammation in the body and heal leaky gut. Food can be life-giving or life-taking. You have the chance to heal your body with every mouthful. Become mindful of what you are eating. Reduce the sugar in your diet! Kick gluten and dairy to the curb! Make over your fat intake! Eat more whole foods! Make sure you eat raw vegetables (think salad) daily! Fill your plate with 75 percent vegetables and 25 percent lean, organic, wild-caught protein, and a small serving of a healthy, starchy carbohydrate like sweet potatoes, quinoa, brown rice, or less sweet fruits.

For breakfast, think vegan protein smoothies or chia seed pudding, or scrambled eggs with spinach. For lunch, think big salad with lots of organic vegetables and olive oil and lemon dressing or avocados instead of oil. For dinner, think small serving of grass-fed beef or organic chicken and a lightly steamed green vegetable like broccoli or Brussel sprouts or asparagus, and a small side of sweet potatoes. Cooking vegetables destroys many of the valuable vitamins so having raw vegetables each day improves your vitamin intake. When cooking them, lightly steam or lightly sauté them to preserve more of the nutrients. Drink water instead of tea or soda. Stay hydrated. Sometimes a salad seems too cooling to the body like in the fall and winter when temperatures fall. We like to add warm vegetable broth or warm bone broth to our salad to make it like a soup but still retain the vital nutrients in the greens.

How can you improve your liver and intestinal function? Consider doing cleanses at the turn of each season. Add raw vegetables and raw, low sugar juices daily. Drink water with lemon juice and add potassium rich foods like sweet potatoes, tomato sauces, beets and beet greens, spinach, beans and coconut water to your diet. Do not overeat! Overeating is toxic to the liver.

Consider taking a digestive enzyme with larger meals to improve digestion. Consider taking a high-quality probiotic to improve good gut bacteria.

CHAPTER 7
Toxic Exposure

"The nation behaves well if it treats its natural resources as assets which it must turn over to the next generation increased, and not impaired, in value."
– Theodore Roosevelt

In our whole-body solution for healing the thyroid, reducing the body's toxic burden is a must. There are many toxins in our environment that have a profound effect on thyroid function. We come in contact with hundreds of chemicals daily that can accumulate and cause damage to the body and significantly affect our health. Everyone is unique. We all have our own genetic tolerance for toxins. We will highlight different genetic weaknesses or SNPs in a later chapter.

We have taught many classes helping people reduce their toxic load by replacing toxic chemicals with cleaner versions or with essential oils. In our classes, we hear stories of how people were never sensitive to something like their shampoo or cleaning products or foods that they ate, and then all of the sudden, bam, they feel as if they are allergic to everything! This is what we call filling your toxic bucket. The size of your toxic bucket is dependent on your genetic makeup, but for most people with hypothyroidism, your bucket is small! Once it fills up, your health is compromised. Damage is occurring all along, but it is only when the toxins have caused enough damage to our health that we take notice of our symptoms. The goal is to clean out that bucket and stop new toxins from coming in.

There is no way to be 100 percent clean. The FDA sets standards for the maximum amounts of chemicals that are allowed in our food and water that would be considered safe for the majority of the people. But what about those that are more sensitive? Financially, it would be impossible to get every chemical out of our food and our water. There are so many chemicals in our environment that exposure to them is inevitable. What we want to do is to reduce exposure and clean up our bodies from the inside out and outside in.

Wouldn't it have been great to have known about these toxins and to have been able to eliminate them early in our lives to prevent disease? Hopefully, what you learn will allow you to help others clean up their toxins and maybe lower the toxic exposure for your children or grandchildren early on to prevent health problems in their future. We will be discussing toxins in the environment, in body care and makeup, in your medicine cabinet, your cleaning products, and in your food and water. We will discuss how they affect the thyroid and how to avoid them.

ENVIRONMENTAL TOXINS

Perchlorates

Do you ever look up in the sky and see all of the vapor trails formed by jets as they are traveling from one place to another? Looks pretty innocent, right? Well, they are not! Rocket fuel (jet fuel) is the major source of perchlorates in our environment and they are released into the air in that very vapor trail. Perchlorate falls to the ground and rainwater washes it into the lakes and streams and rivers and ends up in our drinking water. It can be taken up by our fruits and vegetables. When cows eat the grass they take in perchlorates and it ends up in their milk. When we take this chemical into our bodies mainly by drinking unfiltered water, the perchlorates impact our thyroid glands by blocking the uptake of iodine into the thyroid. The thyroid is the main target for perchlorates. This prevents the synthesis of thyroid hormones. New studies show that much lower levels of perchlorates, that were traditionally considered safe, can be detrimental to the thyroid.

So, what can we do? Even though our drinking water is the cleanest in the world, we still have problems. Filter your water. Go to our website to see the filters we prefer, sandawellnessduo. com.

PCBs

Polychlorinated biphenyls were man-made industrial chemicals whose use was widespread. They were used in manufacturing electrical equipment, in making paints, printing inks, paper, pesticides, hydraulic fluids, and many other products. It was even sprayed on dirt roads or construction sites to reduce dust. These chemicals were banned in 1979 when they were thought to have an unintended impact on human and environmental health. Since then, PCBs have been shown to cause cancer, have a negative effect on the endocrine, immune, reproductive, and nervous systems.

Since they are synthetic, man-made chemicals, they persist and bioaccumulate in our environment. These chemicals tend to accumulate in fatty areas of the body (as all fat soluble toxins do) and the bodies of animals. PCBs have been found in the fat and liver of humans and in breast milk. We are exposed by eating contaminated fatty meats, fish higher up on the food chain, like tuna, and poultry. PCBs reduce the amount of circulating thyroid hormone by interfering with the enzymes that convert T4 to T3 in the liver.

So what can you do? If you are a meat eater, eat smaller portions and leaner cuts of meat. Eat organic poultry, pasture-raised meats, wild-caught fish. Farm-raised fish have higher amounts of toxins including PCBs. Avoid fish higher on the food chain, like tuna and farm-raised fish. Plants have the lowest amounts of PCBs.

BPA

Bisphenol-A is used in the manufacturing of plastics including the lining of food cans, dental sealants, and polycarbonate plastics. BPA is so prevalent that it can be found in the blood of pregnant women, in amniotic fluid, and in the umbilical cord and placenta and other body tissues. BPA specifically binds to thyroid receptors directly inhibiting the activity of T3 on the cell. When thyroid testing shows T3 in the normal range and you are still having hypothyroid symptoms, BPA could be adding to the cause. Scientists estimate that over 80 percent of people tested have measurable BPA in their bloodstream. BPA also interferes with the adiponectin, a hormone that is produced by fat tissue and increases fat metabolism and insulin sensitivity. Interestingly, adiponectin is significantly lower in hypothyroid patients making it harder to lose weight. Known as an estrogen mimic, BPA increases estrogen in the body possibly leading to problems caused by excess estrogens.

BPA has been replaced with BPS that was thought not to leach, but recent studies show that it leaks and now is detectable in 81 percent of Americans and can have the same effect as BPA.

So what can we do? Ditch the plastics folks! Use glass or stainless steel. Never heat in plastic because more of the BPA and BPS gets into the food. Never leave plastic water bottles in a hot car. Look for BPA free cans of food but even better would be to use fresh or frozen foods instead of canned foods.

Pesticides

A non-profit group, Beyond Pesticides, found that there are at least 60 pesticides used today that have shown to affect the thyroid gland's ability to produce T4 and T3. Insecticides and fungicides have also been implicated. If you have ever noticed organic vegetables have a shorter refrigerator life than conventional vegetables, it's because of the antifungals sprayed on them to prolong their shelf life. These are thyroid disrupting.

So what can we do? When possible, buy all organic! Go to our website to get a list of the *Dirty Dozen* and the *Clean 15* to guide you as you shop for cleanest foods. You will see which ones to buy organic and which are okay to buy conventionally. Wash your fruits and vegetables in a vegetable wash before consuming.

Halogen

Fluorine, chlorine, bromine, and iodine are all halogens that we come in contact with daily. The thyroid only uses iodine to make thyroid hormone. The halogens fluorine, chlorine, and bromine will compete with iodine for entry into the thyroid. They block the iodine receptors so thyroid hormone cannot be produced. Chlorine can interfere with conversion of T4 to T3. We come in contact with chlorine primarily in our water and in our cleaning products. When you shower or swim in a pool, chlorine goes directly into your bloodstream. Bromine can be found in breads and flour products, lemon-lime flavored drinks (brominated vegetable oil), and cough and cold medications. Fluoride is found in toothpaste and drinking water.

So what can we do? Use a shower filter to limit your exposure. Use a water filter that filters out halogens. On our website we have the ones we use posted. We are eliminating breads and sodas so that source will not be a problem. Use therapeutic essential oils when you feel sick before you reach for the cold medicine. Use a toothpaste free of fluoride and SLS (sodium lauryl sulfate).

Mercury and Other Heavy Metals

Mercury is such an interesting metal. It's super shiny and has a high surface tension that allows it to make rounded beads. It is the only liquid metal and can turn into a vapor when exposed to the air. Mercury is very toxic! When mercury gets into your body, it is absorbed by the thyroid where it is stored. It prevents iodine from getting in the cell to make thyroid hormone. One hypothesis about the way Hashimoto's develops is an accumulation of mercury in the thyroid and the body's immune system mounts a response attacking the thyroid in an effort to get rid of the invader, mercury. Mercury is very hard to get it out of your body, and as long as it is there, you will have lower thyroid function.

How are we exposed to mercury? The biggest source comes from coal burning power plants. Coal has mercury impurities in it and when burned, the mercury gets into the air and drifts in the wind and settles to the ground. Coal burning emits over 70,000 pounds of mercury into the air each year. When it rains, rainwater is washed into the lakes and streams and rivers (like many other toxins) and eventually winds up in our drinking water. Our municipal water suppliers are required by law to reduce mercury to a level of 2ppb or.002mg/L, but trace amounts add up.

Another source are silver dental amalgams of yesteryear that are still in our baby boomers! They are made out of mercury, and slowly over time, they vaporize in your mouth and get into your body and are absorbed mainly by the thyroid. Mercury is found in some vaccines and has been a source of mercury for many years. It can be found in cosmetics and pesticides.

It bioaccumulates in animals so the ones on top of the food chain are the ones most contaminated, like tuna, farm-raised fish, bluefish, grouper, sea bass, and shark. Trace amounts add up over time in our bodies.

Other metals that affect the body are lead and aluminum. Lead is present in the air that we breathe, in old paints, in our water, and can get into our bodies and wreak havoc. It accumulates and replaces the calcium in our bones and leads to osteoporosis. It is released slowly from the bones into our bloodstream and damages other soft tissues of the body.

Aluminum exposure comes from the air and water, our pots and pans, in processed foods we eat, in aluminum foil, antiperspirants, medications, and vaccines. It accumulates in our bodies over time and can be found in breast tissue and in the brain. Some studies suggest that excess aluminum can contribute to Alzheimer's disease and breast cancer, osteoporosis, autism in newborns, and can damage the central nervous system. It acts as an estrogen mimic leading to hormone imbalances including hypothyroidism.

So what can we do? We will be talking about how we are detoxifying these metals in chapter ten on genetics. This has greatly reduced our heavy metal burden. Have your amalgams removed by a dentist that understands and has been trained on the proper way to remove these. (Susan: *I believe that this was my trigger. I had them removed as soon as the information was coming out about how amalgams could damage your health but my dentist was not trained properly. As he was taking them out, I was swallowing the debris and breathing in the vapor. Shortly after this, I started showing symptoms of hypothyroidism.*)

Soy

Soy inhibits thyroid peroxidase that inhibits the thyroid's ability to use iodine, reducing the amount of thyroid hormone made. It disrupts the conversion of T4 to T3 in the tissues like the muscle. It has been shown that infants fed soy formula had a prolonged increase in their TSH levels compared to infants fed non-soy formulas. This would indicate a degree of hypothyroidism.

So what can we do? Avoid soy in all forms. Much of the soy out there is genetically modified and not healthful. Read labels to avoid soy. (Anna: *I believe that this could have been one of my triggers. I was fed soy formula because I was intolerant to cow's milk formula. It wasn't known to have this effect back then.*)

Toxins in Body Care Products and Makeup

We do not think about the skin as an organ but in fact, it is the largest organ in the body. It's easy to slather on skin care lotions and potions without thinking about how these products might impact your health. You might not know that these ingredients can be absorbed through the skin and add to your toxic burden. The skin is a sponge! Many chemical ingredients in skin care products are found to be endocrine disruptors. Endocrine disruptors interfere with the way normal hormones function, often blocking the receptors for hormone attachment.

Count the number of products you use each day, from your shampoo and body wash to your lotions and skin care regimen to your hair care products. How many do you use? According to the Environmental Working Group, the average woman uses 12 personal care products containing 168 unique ingredients. In Europe, 1,300 synthetic ingredients have been banned due to their possible adverse effect on health. In the U.S., we have only banned eight and restricted three of those ingredients. It's left to the consumer to know what is safe. Buyer beware!

The beauty industry is highly unregulated. You'd think the FDA would do a better job of regulating this industry—but it doesn't. How do these chemicals react with each other once they are inside the bloodstream? No one knows the real effect. There are many chemicals in products that add to our toxic burden, but we will discuss those that are known to affect thyroid function. Read your labels for these and move to safer products.

Parabens (Methylparaben, Butylparaben, Propylparaben, etc.)
Parabens are used as preservatives that prevent the growth of bacteria and mold in cosmetics. Sounds important, right? Not so much! Parabens have been detected in breast tumor tissue and are known to act as an estrogen mimic, increasing the risk of breast cancer. Parabens are found in many personal care products like shampoos, body washes, deodorants, makeup, facial cleansers, and they are also found in pharmaceuticals and foods. Studies have shown a correlation between lower circulating thyroid hormone levels in adults with high paraben levels.

So what can we do? Read ingredient labels and avoid all parabens.

Fragrance
Have you noticed the increase in the number of fragrances in products today? Just a stroll down the cleaner and detergent

isle in the grocery store and you will be amazed with all of the different fragrances you encounter. We all want to smell good, but synthetic fragrances are not the way to go. Look for the word fragrance or perfume in the ingredients list of the products you are using. The word fragrance gives manufacturers a place to protect their secret formula and those ingredients do not have to be disclosed to the consumer. There are over 3,000 different chemicals that a manufacturer can pick and choose from until they get just the right combination of chemicals for the fragrance they are looking for to be in their products. They don't have to list the ones they choose in making up their unique formula. Fragrances can contain a number of endocrine disrupting chemicals which depress thyroid function.

Synthetic fragrance is the second most common cause of allergy that send patients to their dermatologist with rashes and hives. Fragrance triggers respiratory allergies, headaches/migraines, burning eyes, and asthma attacks. Ingredients in fragrances have been associated with cancer and neurotoxicity.

According to a 1986 report by the National Academy of Sciences, 95 percent of the ingredients used to produce synthetic fragrances are derived from petroleum and include carcinogenic benzene derivatives, aldehydes and toluene, and many other chemicals linked to cancer and birth defects. The EPA found that synthetic fragrances were often shown to contain hormone disruptors. So, ditch the fragrances from your body care products, cleaning products, laundry products, and air fresheners.

So what can we do? Try using high quality, essential oils instead. Essential oils are the volatile extracts from plants. Have you ever rubbed rosemary between your hands and smelled the aroma left behind, or smelled the lemon essence when you were zesting the peel for a recipe? These are essential oils. Essential oils are what makes herbs healthful.

However, labels can be confusing. There is lavender essential oil, and there is lavender fragrance oil. Lavender fragrance oils are synthetic and do not offer the same benefits as lavender essential oil. You will find the fragrance oils in cleaning products and body care products. They offer no therapeutic benefit, even though they may claim that they have the same benefit as the essential oil. Essential oils are expensive and usually not used in cheaper products. If it is a real essential oil, the label will include its common name and its scientific name, like peppermint (mentha piperita).

There is such a difference in the quality of essential oils on the market today because they are beginning to be all the rage! Many companies buy their essential oil from wholesalers, but they have no idea where the oil was derived or how it was distilled. They just add their label to the essential oil and sell it as their own. Many of these oils have little to no therapeutic value. Many are adulterated with cheaper oils and filler oils. We can help you decide which ones are therapeutic and worth the money. We have a webinar on how to begin using essential oils if you'd like to learn more. Contact us at sandawellnessduo@gmail.com and we will send you some information! We will teach you how to get started!

Phthalates

Phthalates are a group of compounds that are added to products to increase flexibility and softness of plastics. The main phthalates used in cosmetics and personal care products are dibutyl phthalate in nail polish, diethyl phthalate in perfumes and fragrances, and dimethyl phthalate in hairspray. These are all known to be endocrine disruptors and have been linked to increased risk of breast cancer, early breast development in girls, and reproductive birth defects in males and females. Phthalates are associated with lower serum levels of T4 and T3 and an elevated TSH. Unfortunately, it is not disclosed on the product if it's added to the fragrance. It is added to enhance the "staying power" of the fragrance to help it linger.

So what can we do? Avoid fragrances in your products. Add your own essential oils to body products. We will show you how!

Triclosan and Triclocarban
These are used as antimicrobial agents in soaps and toothpastes, dish detergents, and deodorants. They are known endocrine disruptors, especially affecting the thyroid and reproductive hormones. They irritate the skin and contribute to making bacteria antibiotic resistant.

So what do we do? Avoid triclosan by reading your labels. Using soap and water to wash your hands has been shown to be just as effective as using hand sanitizers with triclosan. Avoid triclosan in laundry soaps, dish detergents, hand washes and sanitizers, and toothpaste.

Sodium Lauryl Sulfate (SLS) / Sodium Laureth Sulfate (SLES)
These are surfactants and can be found in over 90 percent of personal care products. They help the product foam and be

sudsy. SLSs are known to be skin, lung, and eye irritants. These can be found in shampoo, shower gels, and facial cleansers and can also be found in household cleaning products. They are suspected to damage the skin's immune system causing inflammation. We have heard people say that they don't feel clean if their shampoo or soap doesn't suds up. But there is a cost for the suds.

So what can we do? Read labels and avoid SLS!

Chemical Sunscreens (Retinyl, Palmitate, Oxybenzone, and Octyl Methozycinnamate, Benzophenone)

These sunscreens are found in many personal care product like lip balms and foundation makeup. They have been found to have hormone disrupting effects. They can block thyroid receptors and inhibit the activity of thyroid peroxidase, the enzyme involved in making thyroid hormone.

So what can we do? Look for mineral-based sunscreens. Wear materials that block UV rays. Use an umbrella at the beach. Avoid prime UVA, UVB hours between 11:00 a.m. – 2:00 p.m.

There are so many other chemicals that add to our body's toxic burden but these are specific to the thyroid. Avoid all synthetic chemicals in body care products and makeup.

Toxins in Cleaning Products

What makes you think your house is clean? Most people answer, "The way it smells!" We have already talked extensively about the dangers of fragrance in your body care products, but the same holds true with cleaning products. Fragrance is unregulated. Did you know that the inside of your house can be more toxic than the outside? Fragrance adds to that pollution. Scented candles and plugins and dryer sheets are so toxic to our bodies and interfere with thyroid function and the function of other endocrine glands.

The average household uses cleaning products that contain 62 known toxins. Fragrance is right up there on the list. Other ingredients might not directly affect the thyroid but do add to your toxic bucket. There are other chemicals that add to our toxic burden that are present in cleaning products, but that list is long and for another book! By cleaning up your products, you will eliminate many of those as well. We can help you to start to reduce the toxins in your home that can be making you sick. Go to our Thank You page for information on making over your cleaning products.

So what can we do? Use a diffuser to diffuse essential oils that actually clean the air of pollutants. Make your own cleaning products with essential oils or find cleaner versions of your products. Use wool dryer balls with essential oils dropped on them in your dryer instead of dryer sheets.

Toxins in Your Medicine Cabinet

Some medications are necessary but as your body begins to function better and you start cleaning up your body's toxic burden, it's possible for the need of those medicines to decrease. Synthetic medications are not recognized by the body in the way natural ingredients are. Synthetics have to be metabolized by the liver and many times the liver doesn't know what to do with that synthetic, so it stashes it away in your fat tissue. Just like synthetic chemicals bioaccumulate in the fat of animals, they do the same thing to us. The fat in our bodies are a storehouse for toxins. As we lose the fat, we lose some of that toxic burden. Our bodies began to work better and we feel more energized. Our moods improve. We have the energy to get through our day, and maybe get to the gym and to look after the ones we love.

There are many of your over the counter preparations that can be replaced with certified pure, therapeutic grade essential oils and supplements. Medicines are the only chemicals that are allowed to say they "cure" an ailment or a disease. (But do they really do that?) Food, essential oils, supplements cannot be marketed as a "cure" or a "treatment" for any condition that there is a medication for already on the market. That law is in place to protect the consumer against fraudulent claims of miracle cures. However, there are many things that you can do and use instead of first turning to an OTC drug that only adds to your toxic burden or interferes with the digestive process and gut bacteria.

Neal came to us looking for an alternative treatment he could use for his breathing conditions. He told us he had been on medication for 25 years which included an emergency inhaler and a steroid inhaler to suppress his immune system. He was never far from his emergency inhaler and if he ever forgot to take his steroid inhaler in the morning, he would leave work and go home to take it. He had a couple of sinus infections every year due to suppressing his immune system. Anna and I introduced him to certified pure, therapeutic grade essential oils and told him to give them a try as a supplement to what he was already using. We told him how cleaning up his diet would help as well. He told us after using the oils we suggested, he was able to get off of his emergency inhaler and his steroid. He has not had a sinus infection in the four years since he started using essential oils. He has used his emergency inhaler only a few times since then as well. He said he is sold on using these essential oils to help with his breathing problems!

Remember that we are making no claims to diagnosis, treat, cure, or prevent any disease.

CHAPTER 8

Sleep and Stress

"Our anxiety does not empty tomorrow of its sorrow but only empties today of its strengths."

– Charles H. Spurgeon

How well did you sleep last night? How well do you sleep most nights? Sleep is one of the most restorative things you can do for your body! It helps the body repair itself and resets your hormones. It lowers cortisol, insulin, and leptin, and increases melatonin, human growth hormone (HGH) and testosterone. Sleep is the ultimate anti-ager! If you want to lose weight and heal your body, sleep needs to be a priority. How do these hormones mentioned affect sleep and how is sleep connected to stress? How are sleep and stress connected to weight loss?

A good night's sleep lowers cortisol, your body's stress hormone involved in the fight or flight response. When your body senses stress, cortisol is released and there is a cascade of events that occur in your body. Once the stress is resolved, cortisol and the other hormones released in response, go back to normal. On a daily basis, the pituitary and the hypothalamus are at work monitoring the levels of cortisol in the blood.

Too much stress or chronic stress causes the levels of cortisol to get out of whack and cortisol levels remain higher than normal, making sleep seem almost impossible. A good night's sleep reduces cortisol levels helping you to be able to better handle stressful situations that may come up during the day. But how can you restore your ability to sleep? Keep reading!

Sleep lowers leptin, the appetite regulator. It is hard to think about healthy food when you are tired. Carbohydrates will be the food you crave to try to increase your energy. A good night's sleep will help you make better food choices instead of scarfing down the donuts in the breakroom at work.

Sleep increases melatonin. Melatonin is secreted by the pineal gland in the brain and regulates your body's circadian rhythm. It is often called the sleep hormone by inducing sleep at night, but research is showing it does so much more. It also acts as a powerful antioxidant and anti-inflammatory and it's shown to boost immunity.

Sleep increases human growth hormone. HGH is vital in keeping lean muscle mass on the body and to increase fat burning, enhancing weight loss. It plays a vital role in cell regeneration, growth and repair of tissues, and stimulates collagen synthesis! Going to bed by 10:00 p.m. allows more of it to be secreted. A good workout plan also increases HGH, which you will learn about in chapter nine on exercise.

Testosterone (yes, women secrete small amounts of testosterone) aids in burning fat, building muscle, increasing bone density, and improving sex drive.

Estrogen and progesterone also play important roles in sleep. Low levels of estrogen cause hot flashes which can keep you up at night and can prevent you from being able to fall asleep. Low progesterone levels cause you to have a greater risk of experiencing anxiety and a worried mind, making it hard to fall asleep. It's the wired but tired scenario.

Why is it that many people with hypothyroidism have such a hard time with sleep? Either they can't get to sleep or they sleep so lightly that the sleep they do get is not restful; or on the flip side, they can get to sleep but can't seem to get out of bed in the morning and when they do finally get up, they feel sluggish. Let's explore!

THE MELATONIN–CORTISOL CYCLE

Normally, there is a natural cycle that allows for sleep and wakefulness. It's called the melatonin-cortisol cycle. Cortisol starts to rise in the morning to wake you up. It keeps you awake during the day and decreases gradually throughout the day as melatonin gradually starts to rise. When it gets dark more melatonin is secreted and you begin to get sleepy somewhere around 9-9:30 p.m. Bright lights at night, like light coming from your computer or the television, can prevent melatonin from being secreted.

What happens to this cycle with hypothyroidism? The thyroid is intimately connected to the adrenals. The adrenals produce cortisol. Cortisol is released in response to stress and low blood sugar. When cortisol is overproduced, as would be in the case of chronic stress, TSH levels decline, reducing the amount of thyroid hormone produced by the thyroid. It also inhibits T4 to T3 conversion in your tissues and causes a rise in reverse T3 (RT3), favoring D3 over D1. So when the adrenal function is elevated, thyroid function is suppressed. In addition, chronically elevated cortisol leads to a suppression of melatonin, so sleep evades you.

To add to the problem, there is another process at play. It's called *pregnenolone steal!* Our sex organs make the majority of our sex hormones, but the adrenals make enough sex hormones to keep these hormones in the normal range. It's an important player in sex hormone levels in the body.

PREGNENOLONE STEAL

Pregnenolone is a steroidal hormone produced mainly in the adrenal glands from cholesterol. It is the precursor, from which nearly all other hormones are produced, including DHEA, progesterone, testosterone, estrogen, and cortisol. When you are healthy, pregnenolone keeps energy levels high, and elevates overall mental acuity and mood, and maintains normal hormone levels. In addition to improving mood, it also boosts the immune system, maintains skin health, maintains the sleep cycle, helps the body have a healthy stress response, and aids in fertility.

When your adrenals are stressed, pregnenolone levels will drop. There are many causes of adrenal stress. There is emotional stress, stress from inadequate or inappropriate exercise, stress from poor nutrition and increased insulin levels, stress from high levels of inflammation, stress from aging, and stress from not being physically active.

Another big factor in pregnenolone levels are thyroid hormone levels. When your thyroid hormones are low, the adrenals have to pick up the slack, and they do that by producing more cortisol and adrenalin to keep the body going. You've heard of running on adrenalin? Your body is actually running on adrenalin and cortisol instead of thyroid hormones. After a period of time, the adrenals become fatigued. This is what happens when you are under chronic stress.

What happens to your sex hormones? When the body perceives stress, more of the pregnenolone is pushed into producing more cortisol to keep the body going and less goes into making the sex hormones, hence, pregnenolone steal. This lowers the levels of testosterone, estrogen and progesterone. This interferes with sleep due to higher levels of cortisol. It interferes with fertility and libido due to decreased sex hormones. It interferes with fat burning and weight loss due to lower thyroid function.

HOW CAN YOU REVERSE PREGNENOLONE STEAL?

Important tips on how to reverse pregnenolone steal is to reduce inflammation, reduce stress, and improve sleep. We are cleaning up diet and toxic load and toxic thoughts to reduce inflammation, and we will talk more in chapter 10 on genetics about other ways we are reducing inflammation and have had amazing results. Lowering inflammation decreases stress on the body and helps improve pregnenolone levels.

So what about sleep and stress? Sleep lowers stress, and decreasing stress improves sleep! Which one comes first? It's kind of like which came first, the chicken or the egg? Have you ever been told by your doctor to reduce stress and to get more sleep, and maybe they gave you an antidepressant and a sleep aid thinking that would solve the problem. But in the long run, it doesn't.

Susan: *I had trouble with insomnia for many years. Even when I started thyroid medication, my sleep did not improve much. I had a hard time going to sleep, and when I did fall asleep, the slightest noise or light from my alarm clock woke me up. I was irritable, I became angry easily, and I'd blow up when I was confronted with someone who disagreed with me. It was terrible! I didn't want to be this way. It was a combination of inflammation, stress, toxins, and everything we have talked about so far.*

Anna: *I have had trouble waking up in the morning for as long as I can remember. Going to sleep was not the problem. I fell asleep easily, but waking up was such a problem for me. When I did wake up, I didn't feel rested. I was sluggish and irritable, and it would take about 30 minutes to get going. I never scheduled 8:00 a.m. classes in college because I knew I wouldn't make it! For me, it was a combination of inflammation, food allergies, and stress, and all of the other things we have talked about.*

SLEEP

How do you improve your sleep without sleeping pills? Improve what is called your sleep hygiene! Here are some things we have done to improve sleep.

1. Make sure your room is dark and cool. Cool the room to around 68 degrees. Remember that in order to produce the maximum amount of melatonin, the room needs to be dark.
2. Have a bedtime ritual like soaking in an Epsom salt bath at night, reading, staying away from bright lights and eating junk food.
3. Limit your daytime naps to 20-30 minutes. These are called power naps. This can reduce your need for caffeine in the afternoon.
4. Avoid caffeine after 5:00 in the afternoon so your body has time to process it. Avoid it totally if you can. Take a power nap instead.
5. Exercising is so important for improved quality of sleep. Try getting a workout in earlier in the day if nighttime workouts interfere with your sleep. Everyone is different, so see what time of the day for workouts works best for you.
6. Avoid alcohol. Alcohol is known to help you fall asleep faster, but too much can disrupt sleep in the second half of the night as your body is processing the alcohol.
7. Get adequate exposure to natural light during the day. It has been shown that exposure to sunlight during the

day, and darkness at night, helps to maintain a healthy sleep-wake cycle.

8. Invest in a sound maker that creates delta waves to help with sleep. Brainwaves are electromagnetic waves produced by the activity in the brain. Research shows that each of our states of consciousness is associated with a specific pattern of brainwave activity. Delta waves are associated with states of deep relaxation and rejuvenating sleep. Avoid using an app on your phone because of the radiofrequencies emitted (RF) could interfere with sleep. Try to limit all electronics next to the bed. Make sure your internet router is not near your bedroom.

9. Try not to eat a heavy, spicy, fatty meal for dinner. This can interfere with digestion and make sleeping more difficult.

10. Drink a cup of tea that improves sleep like Yogi's Bedtime Tea before bed.

11. Diffuse a high quality, therapeutic lavender essential oil in your bedroom to help with relaxation. It can be applied to the back of the neck and on the feet too.

12. Consider high quality supplements like valerian root extract or a magnesium product like Natural Calm to use 30 minutes before bedtime. Magnesium helps your body to relax naturally and so many of us are low in magnesium. Talk with your doctor before adding a hormone like melatonin to your regimen.

STRESS

Here are things that we have done to improve stress.

The number one thing that has improved our response to stress is getting a good workout in several times during the week. Walking is important here, too. We will be talking more about these in chapter nine on exercise.

The things we talked about earlier, like starting a gratitude journal, staying positive, knowing what your goals are, and keeping your mind on the prize instead of letting other people steal your thunder and your passion—all of these practices will lower your stress level. Mediation, deep breathing, and restorative exercise like yoga are also cortisol reducing. Practice self-care. Get a massage or a facial or a long soak in the bath, or something special just for you.

Smile! There is magic in smiling! This little act changes your attitude whether you realize it or not. It raises your self-confidence and increases your happiness. Did you know that by smiling you increase the activity in the left frontal cortex, the region of the brain that controls happiness? When you are frowning, you decrease the activity here so happiness doesn't come. When you are frowning, you are not approachable. You are putting out negative energy, and negative energy returns to you. Smiling increases your vibration and you attract more positive energy—energy begets energy!

There are many essential oils that can be used to improve your mood and reduce your stress. Your nostrils are connected to the limbic system of the brain through the olfactory bulb. The limbic system controls your basic emotions, like pleasure, anger and fear, your perceptions of your environment, your sense of smell, your behavior, and long-term memory. Have you ever smelled something and it took you back to a memory in your past or made you feel a certain way? Our sense of smell is unique compared to our other senses of taste, sight, and hearing, because the sense of smell bypasses parts of the brain that our other senses can't. Aromas goes straight to the brain. Because of this, aromas can often cause immediate and strong emotional reactions that are based on memory.

High quality, therapeutic essential oils can have a dramatic effect on the limbic system. The molecules that make up essential oils are so small that they are able to cross into the brain and have a positive effect on mood, anxiety, anger, depression. They aid in reducing stress by reducing negative emotions.

We have a webinar that you will have access to that will help you learn how to start using essential oils to help reduce your stress and toxic load as a thank you for purchasing our book. Email us at sandawellnessduo@gmail.com and ask us for help.

Reducing stress and improving sleep are vital in your ability to lose weight and keep it off and live vibrantly.

CHAPTER 9

Exercise

*"It is a shame for a woman to grow old without ever seeing
the strength and beauty of which her body is capable."*
– Socrates

W e are bombarded with images of perfectly shaped, sexy bodies in the media. We fall into the trap of thinking that this is what our bodies are supposed to look like; toned to a tee, no cellulite, a tight butt, no under eye circles, impeccable skin. But is this reality? What they don't tell you is that the pictures are airbrushed and enhanced before printing. And that celebrity that just lost all of that baby weight had personal trainers, a personal chef, and stylists at her beck and call, and she still needs airbrushing and enhancing.

A chef on television who has a perfect body admits that she does not eat all of the pasta she prepares on her show, and she only eats it occasionally and that her diet is actually filled with salads and fresh vegetables. What about the chef that says everything is better with butter, while not disclosing that she had developed diabetes and had to change her diet but, rather, alluding to her fans that she was eating this way and suggesting that this kind of cooking was healthy? Not to mention the celebrities that down alcohol as if it were water making you think that this is okay. Why does the media deceive us? Where is the responsibility?

What about the supplement companies out there that promise you'll lose weight drinking this magic coffee or taking this magic pill? Nothing comes that easy. It is a waste of money.

We can't leave out those infomercials with those perfectly toned fitness models working on a piece of equipment implying that this is all you need to have that ripped body, toned legs and perfect arms in just a few minutes a day. What about all of those programs that promise you the body you so desperately want if you buy their product? They make it seem so simple.

We try to recreate the workouts we see on reality weight loss shows and think that we have to run insane amounts of miles for those long, lean legs or log hours at the gym lifting weights and climbing the stair stepper, meanwhile, drastically cutting calories to achieve that beach body we all want. This is the wrong approach. The fact is 95 percent of people who go on crash diets and have unrealistic workout plans that can't be maintained long term, end up gaining all of it back, and 66 percent of those people end up fatter than they were before they started. Not the outcome we signed up for.

If you have been going about exercise in this way, you could be harming your metabolism and causing more long-term damage than you realize. In a world looking for the quick fix and instant gratification, overindulging in exercise and crash dieting are not uncommon things. This could be the reason you are not seeing those results you are working so hard for.

Having an active lifestyle is so important for our health. If you don't exercise, your muscles lose their tone and become flabby and weak. Your heart becomes fatty and high blood pressure may result. The lungs won't be able to inflate as well and you become winded when you walk up the stairs. Your joints will become stiff and your muscles will tighten. Research shows that inactivity poses as much of a health risk as smoking. Our bodies were not made to sit for long periods of time. Our bodies want to move and be active. As we settle into our adult lives with a family and career, our time for exercising usually gets thrown to the back burner. Sarcopenia is the loss of muscle tissue as a natural part of the aging process. This process can begin to happen as early as your 30s! Physically inactive people can lose 3 to 5 percent of muscle mass with each decade after 30, while physically active people will lose some muscle mass, just not as drastically. Having an active lifestyle should be a top priority to healthy aging.

Physical fitness reduces the chances of developing heart disease, diabetes, and obesity, and also improves your appearance and delays aging. Exercise improves your stamina and strength. Being physically fit allows you to move into your golden years without the chronic diseases that plague so many of our elderly. It all starts when you are younger. Let exercise be a part of your lifestyle.

In order to understand how to lose weight and keep it off, you need to understand what controls your metabolism. From this point on, we will talk about fat loss instead of weight loss, because what we really want is to lose the fat and build muscle to get the body shape that we desire. Have you seen people that go on diets and lose a lot of weight, but their body looks like a smaller, pudgy version of their previous self with no definition? That pudgy body isn't stronger and will not be an efficient fat burner, and they will probably end up regaining some, if not all, of the weight back. We want to change our shape, lose fat, have toned muscles, and be stronger and healthier.

In order to burn fat, we need to understand two important enzymes; hormone sensitive lipase and lipoprotein lipase.

HORMONE SENSITIVE LIPASE

Hormone sensitive lipase is an enzyme that promotes fat burning. It seems like a magic potion that turns on fat burning by breaking apart the fat stored in the fat cells and mobilizing it to be burned. The level of HSL in your body is influenced by the amount of insulin circulating in the blood. The more insulin in the blood, the lower the HSL, hence, less fat burning and more fat storing. In order to burn fat and keep it off, insulin must be lowered. If you have a diet high in carbohydrates, full of breads, pastas, sodas, chips and the like, you will have higher insulin and lower HSL, and will tend to store fat.

LIPOPROTEIN LIPASE

Think of lipoprotein lipase as a fat storing enzyme. The fat in your diet, and the sugar that gets converted to fat is taken up by LPL and stored in the fat or adipose tissue all over the body. The more sugar you consume and the more you overeat, the larger the fat cells become.

We want to turn on HSL and turn down LPL. So how do we do this? We have already said that high insulin stimulates LPL and turns down HSL. Stress is another key. When cortisol levels are high, LPL is turned up and HSL is turned down and fat storage results. Controlling insulin and cortisol is a must when considering fat loss. Stress has no calories, but now, we can see how it adds to fat gain. We have talked about how to reduce cortisol by reducing your stress and getting better sleep.

Low thyroid levels also favor LPL over HSL, further exacerbating the problem of fat loss. We've talked about how inflammation reduces thyroid hormone conversion, and we've given you suggestions for lowering inflammation to have better hormone conversion.

Things that will favor and increase HSL and down regulate LPL are increasing catecholamines like adrenalin, and increasing human growth hormone and testosterone. Balancing hormones is an important key in regulating fat loss. We will discuss the kinds of workouts that stimulate these hormones and increase HSL.

HORMONES AT PLAY IN FAT LOSS

Adrenaline is like the igniter that lights the fire to burn fat. With exercise, adrenalin is released and, in turn, causes the release of other hormones like cortisol, human growth hormone, and testosterone and fat burning begins. Avoid high carb foods or sugary drinks before working out so insulin won't spike and block fat burning. You will end up burning the carbohydrates in your blood instead of turning on HSL to promote fat burning.

Cortisol can be good and it can be bad when it comes to fat burning. When cortisol is in the presence of high insulin, then it becomes fat storing. When cortisol is in the presence of testosterone and human growth hormone, it becomes fat burning. You want to do workouts that promote testosterone and HGH.

Insulin in high levels will prevent fat from being released from the fat cells and will promote fat storage. Our diet suggestions will help balance sugar levels and control insulin levels.

Testosterone and human growth hormone are muscle building and fat burning hormones.

Thyroid hormones help to stabilize your metabolism and work with leptin to maintain your body's weight set point. Your set point is the weight your body returns to. An example would be after a holiday of eating, a healthy metabolism will speed up the metabolism to maintain the set point. With hypothyroidism, maintaining weight loss can be a challenge. Controlling leptin can help you develop a new set point for your body. Building muscle is important here, too.

Leptin controls your appetite. It is released from the fat tissue when the body has enough food stored and tells the brain to decrease hunger. Many people have problems with overeating. Overeating causes leptin levels to remain high and eventually the brain does not respond to reduce appetite, and these people continue to over eat which leads to fat storage and the inability to burn fat. This is called leptin resistance. Eating slower and following our suggestions in diet by lowering sugar and eating raw vegetables which are higher in fiber will help control leptin.

MOVEMENT

Let's talk about movement. Movement is so basic but so important to a fat-loss lifestyle. The majority of us are not moving enough on a daily basis. If you have a desk job and are not getting up much during the day but hit the gym to work out after work; that is still considered sedentary. The recommended minimum amount of steps you should be getting is 10,000. Movement raises HSL and will increase fat burning.

Action steps: Get a fitness/step tracker like a Fitbit to track just how much movement you are getting per day. Take the stairs. Walk at lunch on pretty days. It will reduce your stress. Set an alarm on your phone to get up and walk around every hour. Use a standing desk for part of your day.

Anna: *When I first got my Fitbit, I was so shocked to see how little movement I was getting during the day. I had a desk job at the time, and had an hour commute to work, and even longer commute coming home. I worked out during my lunch break, either ran or lifted weights, several days a week, and thought I was getting enough movement. With an eight-hour workday and two hours of driving, I was sitting the majority of those ten hours. The Fitbit is great because it reminds you to get up and move.*

WORKOUTS

If you have hypothyroidism, you may have problems with adrenal fatigue. If you are suffering from adrenal fatigue, intense workouts will stress your adrenals even more. I suggest more restorative exercise until your adrenals are in better shape. Try walking, a restorative yoga class, lower intensity Pilates workouts, but do some form of exercise. Exercise lowers stress which is a contributing factor in adrenal fatigue. Lowering stress lowers cortisol which will aid in fat loss. When you feel ready, move into the other types of workouts suggested.

HIGH INTENSITY INTERVAL TRAINING (HIIT)

HIIT workouts are designed to be shorter, 20 minutes or so, and have more intensity than traditional cardio. There are periods of intense bursts of activity followed by rest periods. This type of workout is great for fat burning because it releases adrenalin, testosterone, HGH, and cortisol, which stimulates HSL. Remember that cortisol in the presence of testosterone and HGH is fat burning. According to the American College of Sports Medicine, just two weeks of HIIT improves your aerobic capacity as much as six to eight weeks of endurance training like long distance running.

HIIT workouts are actually more effective for fat loss and body change due to the intensity factor. When you work out for longer periods of time, your hormone response is different. Longer workouts leave you hungry and exhausted, and can keep you from being consistent. Shorter, more intense workouts create a hormonal environment for a larger calorie after burn without impacting hunger and cravings. This will give you more energy to push harder for that shorter time frame, leaving you satisfied and consistent, and in the end your body will change. I want to teach you how to work out smarter, not longer.

Another advantage to HIIT workouts is a phenomenon called EPOC (Excess Post Exercise Oxygen Consumption). This phenomenon causes the body to have a sustained oxygen deficit that will take longer to pay back after the workout is over. It may take up to 24-36 hours to recover, and in the meantime, your mitochondria are burning up more fat during those 24-36 hours.

WEIGHTLIFTING

HIIT workouts are great at burning fat and you will build some muscle in the process, but your workout program needs to include weightlifting as well. Weight training will help you build muscle, which will in turn, burn more fat. You will be stronger and more confident. Concentrate on upper body muscles on one day and lower body muscles the next. We recommend two to three days of HIIT training and two to three days of weight training per week.

While Linda had been very active for many years, she knew she needed to exercise. For years she tried many programs and different workout places, with and without friends for support, and most of the time, had no results. Linda decided to hire Anna to be her personal trainer and since working with her, she has never seen such great results. Linda has back issues with nerve damage due to scoliosis. Anna was able to find ways to work around those issues with great results. Linda started with low weights on many of the machines in October, and since then has been able to increase the weight on all of them more than she ever thought possible. It truly feels great to be strong. Linda says that working with Anna is the best thing she has done for herself in a very long time. Linda also sees a chiropractor regularly, and he is pleased with her improvements and the fact that currently she has *no* back pain and is more flexible than ever!

CHAPTER 10

Genetics, NRF2 and NRF1 Pathways

"The doctor of the future will give no medicine, but will interest his patients in the care of the human frame, diet and in the cause and prevention of disease."
— **Thomas A. Edison**

You may recall form your high-school biology class that the DNA makes up the chromosomes in the nucleus and holds the blueprint for building and maintaining life. Half of your genetic material came from the father and half came from the mother. Everyone's DNA is unique to them, like a fingerprint.

The DNA is made up of individual genes that hold the recipe for making proteins. The gene is copied and carried out of the nucleus to the ribosome inside the cytoplasm; the liquid portion of the cell. The message is transcribed into a protein, like a hormone, that can travel out of the cell, into the bloodstream. The hormone travels to its target cell and attaches to a receptor on the surface of the cell membrane. It gives the cell instructions on how to act. The protein could be an enzyme that catalyzes reactions inside the cell or it could secrete enzymes into the digestive system to break down food. This is an oversimplification but it serves our purpose.

As the body grows or repairs tissue, the cells are added or replaced with new ones through a process called cell replication. The DNA is copied and each new cell gets a complete set of genetic material. Errors in copying the DNA can occur. Although the body has checks and balances to make sure each copy is accurate, mistakes can get through. These errors are called mutations. These mutations get passed down to other cells as they replicate. Sometimes mutations have no impact on the organism. Sometimes the mutations allow the organism to have a better survival rate. Some can be weakening to the organism, and sometimes of course, a mutation can be lethal.

Genes occur in pairs, one on each chromosome. Most mutations are recessive, meaning that the person has one gene with the mutation and one without, so the mutation has no effect. Sometimes, both genes will be expressed but there will be enough of the good protein produced that it doesn't have much effect. When both parents contribute a recessive gene, the mutation will be expressed.

Somatic mutations, or acquired mutations, can happen during a person's lifetime that are caused by environmental factors like ultraviolet radiation from the sun, or chemicals they come in contact with. This type of mutation could cause cancer in the body.

So mutations happen. You hear people say, "Heart disease runs in my family." Or they say diabetes or cancer runs in their family, or "Everyone in my family is overweight so it's in my DNA." We all have genetic predispositions or weaknesses toward certain diseases, but it is very important to realize that the genetic weaknesses we inherit from our parents do not necessarily determine our fate. Outside of highly genetically determined diseases like Huntington's disease, cystic fibrosis, or Down's syndrome, we can modify the behavior of our genes! You are not destined to get a certain disease that you may have a predisposition for; change your environment now!

One of the best ways to study the impact of genetics and the environment is to look at identical twins. Since they are genetically identical, they have the same genetic predispositions. When twins have different lifestyle and dietary habits, the one with the undesirable habits will gain weight and suffer those lifestyle diseases like diabetes and heart disease, where the thinner twin will not.

The most common genetic mutations or variations to the DNA do not have a strong negative effect, so it remains in the population. These changes are called, SNPs, single nucleotide polymorphisms. They are small changes in one or two nucleotides that make up the gene. Nucleotides are the building blocks of the genes. SNPs are thought to generate different versions of the gene in the population. Most SNPs have no real effect on the health of the person but some do. Research shows some SNPs can predict how you will respond to certain drugs, how effectively you can remove toxins from the body, or if you are more at risk for certain diseases, like heart disease, diabetes, hypothyroidism, cancer, or Alzheimer's disease to name a few.

When genetic testing became available to the public, we were all in! We wanted to find out what made us develop hypothyroidism. We were going to find our solution! What we found was that we didn't have the usual SNPs associated with hypothyroidism and we didn't have the currently known SNPs for autoimmunity. The most impactful SNP that we did have was MTHFR, methylenetetrahydrofolate reductase.

In researching, we found that many people with SNPs for the predisposition for hypothyroidism didn't have hypothyroidism (yet), and some people without the SNPs did have hypothyroidism, as was the case with us. So what gives? Does environment play a bigger role in the development or the expression of genetic SNPs than having the SNP itself? We don't know what we don't know. This is a new area of science and there is much to learn, but it is extremely interesting.

MTHFR

Methylenetetrahydrofolate reductase is an enzyme that is involved in metabolizing vitamin B9, folate (the natural form found in food), and folic acid (the synthetic form found in cheaper vitamin supplements and processed foods) into a useable form, 5-methyltetrahydrofolate. This enzyme is found in our methylation pathway and is vital for detoxification and activation of many proteins in the cell. Sometimes referred to as the B vitamin cycle because this is where all of the B vitamins are used in our bodies. The methylation cycle is involved in making DNA, neurotransmitters, removing toxins, fighting infections, and protecting us from oxidative stress. You often hear of the B vitamins as being the stress vitamins because of their importance in feeling good and having energy.

If your methylation cycle is working properly, you are more likely to feel full of energy, in a good mood, and generally feeling well. If it is not working properly, you will feel tired, depressed, irritable, run-down, susceptible to infections, foggy headed, and just an overall feeling of not being well. (Wait, did we just describe hypothyroidism?)

What is methylation? A methyl group is a functional group that can be added to proteins to change their structure and function. This process is called methylation. Methylation helps the body make important compounds in the body like CoQ10, and it helps to turn genes on or off. It helps the body get rid of all of the toxic compounds we've talked about earlier. Another important toxin would be the toxic amino acid, homocysteine. Homocysteine is converted into the beneficial amino acid, methionine, through methylation. L-Methylfolate adds a methyl group to homocysteine producing methionine. If there is not enough methylfolate, homocysteine will accumulate in the blood, scaring the circulatory system leading to heart disease. You can't feel this happening, but over time, higher levels cause damage. Methionine is necessary to make neurotransmitters, and SAM-e, and your body's natural antioxidant, the powerful detoxifier, Glutathione. So if L-methylfolate is low, these will be low as well.

Get natural folate through your diet by choosing dark green vegetables like broccoli, kale, spinach and berries, especially blueberries. Cooking destroys the delicate folate so making sure you get these kinds of vegetables in their raw form is important. We add a handful of kale or spinach to our smoothies in the morning. Some with Hashimoto's worry about the goitrogens in cruciferous vegetables. It only seems to be a problem if you are low in minerals like iodine and selenium. However, limit your serving of these vegetables in raw form to two cups a day and see how you feel. At other meals lightly sauté them.

MTHFR is thought to be present in 45 percent of the population. People with one bad copy, heterozygous, have a decrease in this enzyme's function by about 40 percent. If you have two bad copies, homozygous, then you have a decrease in function of about 70 percent. This reduces the amount of methylfolate that can be made to reduce homocysteine in the blood and make methionine. This reduces the amount of free radicals that can be cleared from the body by glutathione. Dr. Ben Lynch and Dr. Alan Christianson say that most people with hypothyroidism also have MTHFR and suffer from oxidative damage and a reduced ability to clear the body of toxins, so toxins have a bigger impact than someone without MTHFR. People with hypothyroidism tend to have higher levels of inflammation as a result.

Let's look at a couple of the important proteins produced by the methylation cycle.

SAM-E

S-adenosyl-L-methionine, SAM-e, is involved in over 35 different biochemical processes in the body. It works with another B vitamin, B12, to make important neurotransmitters, dopamine, serotonin, and norepinephrine. It works by slowing the breakdown of these brain chemicals allowing them to work longer, and it speeds up the cell's production of the receptors on the cell's surface for neurotransmitter attachment. With MTHFR, people can have lower levels of these neurotransmitters and suffer from depression, anxiety, ADHD, and other neurological disorders.

GLUTATHIONE—THE MOTHER OF ALL ANTIOXIDANTS!

The body is under constant attack from oxidative stress. Oxidative stress is also referred to as oxidative damage, free radicals, advanced glycation end products (AGEs), or reactive oxygen species (ROS). Oxidative stress, no matter what it's called, is the driver of inflammation, aging and chronic diseases, and cancer. People with MTHFR have lower amounts of glutathione, therefore, they have higher levels of inflammation.

The very oxygen that we breathe in contributes to free radical production as our mitochondria use oxygen to make our energy through cellular respiration. In normal metabolism we create these free radicals, or ROS, that are extremely reactive and will react with tissues, stealing away electrons, in turn, making the tissue a free radical. Then the tissue tries to become stable by reacting with other tissues, and the cycle continues. This causes tissue damage. Our own mitochondria can be damaged in the process, too. The very organelles that produce our energy can be damaged by the free radicals it produces. We will see a decrease in energy and will be fatigued easily. The free radicals can damage the DNA or the skin or the cell membranes or any tissue.

Usually our cells are able to balance free radicals with their own antioxidant system. Some level of free radicals are necessary to stimulate muscle growth and tissue repair. However, when the cell's antioxidant system is overwhelmed by the sheer amount of free radicals, this becomes known as oxidative stress. Over the years, accumulated oxidative damage against our tissues leads to diseases like heart disease, diabetes, hypothyroidism, arthritis, MS, and cancer to name a few.

In addition to free radicals being formed from metabolism, they are also produced from UV radiation from sun exposure, or x-ray exposure, heavy metals, pesticides, cigarette smoking, poor diet, overeating, air pollution, viral infections, stress, lack of sleep, excessive exercise, etc.

Glutathione is often referred to as the body's master antioxidant! It is produced by every cell in the body with the highest concentration of glutathione produced in the liver, making the liver a critical organ for detoxification. It is involved in getting rid of viruses, bacteria, heavy metals, radiation, medications, and free radicals. It is essential to the body's natural defense system. The more free radicals and other toxins that the body has to remove, the more glutathione is depleted and the less you have to clear the body. This is where tissue damage can occur. With MTHFR, you have lower levels to begin with and more tissue damage can result from free radicals.

What are some natural ways to reduce free radicals in the body? Learning what lifestyle and dietary habits are increasing free radical formation is the first step. Look at your lifestyle and diet. We have already talked about the benefits of reducing processed foods while including colorful foods and eating green leafy vegetables that are loaded in antioxidants that will fight free radicals. Reduce the amount of animal protein in your diet, and make sure it is organic free range and wild-caught. Eating organic is important to reduce free radical production. Drinking filtered water and filtering your shower water reduces exposure to chlorine and its by-products. We have talked about reducing toxins in your body care products and your cleaning products. We've examined the importance of reducing stress and getting quality sleep, as well as the importance of an active lifestyle. All of these things reduce the formation of free radicals.

NUTRIGENOMICS

There is a new science on the horizon! It's called *nutrigenomics*! It's the study of how nutrients affect gene expression. There are two approaches to this science. First, to investigate for example, how variations in our genes explain why some people can eat high fat diets and have no effect on cholesterol and others experience the exact opposite. Second, to investigate how nutrients can turn certain genes on or off. For example, identifying compounds like turmeric that turn on genes and help the body detoxify.

NRF2 PATHWAY ACTIVATION

The new buzz in medicine is *Nrf2 pathway activation*. So what is Nrf2? Nrf2 is a protein that is in the cytoplasm of the cell, that when activated, turns on the genes involved in detoxification. We call these genes survival genes or stress response genes. Over 200 genes can be turned on or off depending on how it benefits the cell. Antioxidant genes are turned on and fibrotic genes (think scar tissue) are turned off. As we age, this Nrf2 pathway activation slows down. Toxins accumulate and disease ensues.

Among the heavy hitter antioxidant enzymes that are produced by this lifesaving pathway are the powerhouses, glutathione, super oxide dismutase (SOD), and catalase.

SOD was discovered in 1969 by Dr. Joe McCord and Dr. Irwin Fridovich, who received the Elliot Cresson Medal for their work. SOD is the body's most powerful antioxidant enzyme present in every cell. It plays a critical role in reducing internal inflammation and decreasing pain associated with conditions like arthritis. Glutathione works primarily in the liver and SOD works more in each cell. Remember that the mitochondria break down glucose to make energy for our bodies and consume oxygen in the process of cellular respiration. Without oxygen, we can't make energy, but at the same time, unstable, reactive oxygen molecules are created. These are super oxidants or free radicals we usually refer to as reactive oxygen species (ROS). They are especially toxic because they are extremely reactive and will react and damage tissue around them including the mitochondrion itself. Without the mitochondria there is no energy. SOD is responsible for disarming the rogue oxygen molecule, superoxide. It bonds the oxygen molecule to hydrogen peroxide. Hydrogen peroxide is a byproduct of cellular respiration and is a toxin itself but less toxic than the superoxide formed. But not to worry, the enzyme catalase, along with glutathione, breaks the hydrogen peroxide into simple water and oxygen.

Have you experienced pre-mature graying of the hair? This comes from not having enough catalase and glutathione to break down the hydrogen peroxide. Not having enough SOD causes the destruction of the mitochondria and the diseases associated with mitochondrial dysfunction. Researchers are finding that lower levels of SOD and total cell produced antioxidant status may play a larger role in the development of atherosclerosis than elevated total cholesterol, and increase the chance of developing diseases like stroke and Alzheimer's.

So what can we do to ensure we have enough of these antioxidant enzymes produced by our own cells? As we've already discussed, cleaning up our diet and lifestyle, will help our bodies to function better and reduce the chance of disease by reducing inflammation. Get your antioxidants from your foods! Brightly colored, raw salads are great ways to get your antioxidants. Again, cooking will destroy many of the valuable nutrients so make sure some of your vegetables are uncooked or lightly steamed or sautéed. Don't run out and buy glutathione or SOD in supplement form, because they are proteins and they are digested by the digestive system and do no good! Even the expensive liposomal forms are still not well absorbed because they are large molecules.

You will be seeing more about Nrf2 activation as pharmaceutical companies are jumping on the bandwagon to make a drug that can stimulate this pathway.

NRF2 SUPPLEMENTATION

What if there were a supplement that could stimulate your body's on Nrf2 protein that would turn on its own antioxidant enzymes? When you take antioxidant supplements, or eat antioxidants in foods, those antioxidants fight free radicals on a one to one ratio, one antioxidant molecule to one free radical. One and done! If you turn on your own body's ability to produce glutathione, catalase and SOD, and the other 200 or so enzymes, your body fights free radicals at one million to one! How amazing would that be?

There is a supplement that does just that! This supplement is patented and has 23 peer reviewed studies on PubMed, the government's repository for scientific research. No one else can use this combination of natural ingredients to make an Nrf2 activator. It contains the purest forms of turmeric, bacopa, ashwaganda, green tea, and milk thistle. The ingredients work in synergy, meaning they work better together than any of them work on their own. It's not considered an antioxidant but a Nrf2 activator. Dr. McCord worked for 45 years developing this product. It has been found to increase glutathione by 300 percent, SOD by 30 percent, and catalase by 54 percent. It reduces inflammatory markers by 40 percent in 30 days. It has been shown to be so much more effective at reducing free radicals than supplementation with antioxidants.

In addition to a healthy diet and lifestyle, many with hypothyroidism and MTHFR need extra help in reducing toxins to improve health. We have a webinar available to you so that you can see if this would be something that you would like to add to your protocol for improving your health and thyroid function. Just look at the Thank You page for information on how to get this webinar.

We were introduced to this supplement a year and a half ago, and we have had amazing results!

Susan: *My CRP (a measure for inflammation) is finally in a normal range after being high for many years. My heavy metals are clearing from my body. My joints don't hurt. I am more flexible. I am not as sensitive to certain food. My hearing is better. My hearing improved in only two weeks of being on this supplement. Inflammation had caused me to start to lose hearing. It wasn't nerve damage but hearing loss due to inflammation causing my ear bones to start calcifying. Once I started taking this I was stunned when I could actually hear the background music in my favorite restaurant or hear the blinker in the car. I will never be without this supplement.*

Anna: *Having hypothyroidism, I tended to gain fluid, especially around my ankles. Taking this supplement has helped me lose the fluid. I accidently went off of this for a month and my ankles were swollen enough that I couldn't get my boots on. When I got my supplement in the mail the next month, I realized I had not been taking it and started back again, and within a few days, my ankles were back to normal. It has also helped me reduce my thyroid antibodies.*

NRF1—NUCLEAR RESPIRATORY FACTOR 1

Remember we discussed how the mitochondria can be damaged rendering them nonfunctional with high levels of free radicals, ROS. The mitochondria have their own DNA and can regenerate or replicate on their own without the control of the nucleus. When you lift weights, you get stronger because the mitochondria reproduce themselves to make the muscle have more energy to lift heavier. You become stronger. As we age and as inflammation increases, our mitochondria become less efficient at reproducing and our energy declines, and when our bodies age, diseases can begin to take hold. Many researchers say that along with inflammation caused by free radicals, mitochondrial dysfunction is the leading cause of chronic diseases. So both Nrf2 and Nrf1 need to be stimulated to promote healthy aging. Exercising is one way to induce mitochondrial biogenesis or replication. We can also take a product that increases mitochondrial biogenesis to aid in energy production.

Like Nrf2, Nrf1 is beginning to get the attention of medical researchers. You will be hearing more about these two pathways and their abilities to support healthy aging. Let us be your guide to getting the best health possible! Contact us at sandawellnessduo@gmail.com for more information.

CHAPTER 11

Overcoming Obstacles

"The difference between the impossible and the possible lies in a person's determination."

– Tommy Lasorda

At this point, you may be feeling like, *all of this is really good information, but I am too busy to try to implement any of this into my life!* You may be thinking that this is useless and settling for the plot you think you've been given in life would be the easiest thing to do, so you throw up your hands to surrender. If you do this, you will never see improvements in your health.

You may be feeling that you do not have the energy to work out or cook your meals and that you have a hard time just going to work and looking after your family. Trust us when we tell you that when you fill your body with the proper nutrients, your body will respond and you will be filled with so much more energy to do the things you need to do.

Realize that lifestyle changes and changes to your diet are the hardest changes to make. Practicing makes it become a healthful habit. Take things one step at the time. Create a timeline of when you would like to implement these suggestions. Make a list of the most important things you want to work on first. Get that down. Then, make a list for next month and then the next month, until you have implemented the suggestions in this book. Acknowledge where you are today and remember that this is a journey to your new self! Love the process. Be patient with yourself.

Let's look at some strategies for the obstacles you might encounter and find a way to circumvent the urge to give up.

MINDFULNESS

We have talked a good bit about mindfulness and negativity. We want to talk about mindfulness in terms of how negativity impacts your personal energy. It takes energy of mind and body to be mentally prepared to make changes in your lifestyle and diet that lead to a change in your body and your health. Negative emotions zap mental and physical energy.

Think about the last time you had a negative emotion that maybe came from something someone said or did or something you read, that sent your brain spiraling with feelings of anger or feelings of inadequacy or doubt. How long did you think and re-think about that situation? Was it a half of a day? Was it a week? A month? You are still thinking about it? Now imagine the amount of mental energy that you have used thinking about that situation. It has probably been a total waste of time.

Loss of mental energy leads to a loss of physical energy. Remember during those times that you allowed your brain to spiral with emotions; did you have the energy to work out or grab a salad for lunch, cook a good meal, or spend time with your kids or loved ones in a productive way? Did you lash out? Did tasks go unaccomplished?

The way you respond to negative emotions will determine the amount of energy you have to devote to changing your lifestyle and diet. Choosing to acknowledge that emotion and deciding to not let it run your mind is the first step to having energy to do more important things. When that negative emotion comes up, take ten minutes to practice deep breathing and meditation, focusing on your breath instead of the emotion. Repeat your mantra to yourself, and think of happy thoughts and happy places. You will be surprised at the amount of positive energy you will gain from this exercise. You will lower your stress and anxiety. Meditation is something that takes practice but keep with it. Your body will reap the benefits.

TIME MANAGEMENT

Is having no time your excuse for not doing the things necessary for body change? Is a busy work schedule or having small children your excuse of the day? It is often said that you make time for doing things that are important to you. You make time to watch your favorite shows on television. You make time to scroll on Facebook or check your emails. Finding time in a busy schedule is a must.

SOCIAL MEDIA AND TELEVISION TIME

How many social media platforms do you have? How many times a day do you open up those sites to see what's going on? Scrolling on your social media platforms can send you down that rabbit hole of wasted time. Limit the time you spend on social media. Allow yourself time, maybe in the morning and in the evening, to open up these and give yourself a time limit. Set you alarm on your phone so you will be aware of the time.

Stop following negative groups or negative people. Trim your group and friend list. Add posts that are positive uplifting to people. Add value to the friends that follow you. Refrain from posting negative status updates or controversial topics that can lead to negative comments. According to researchers, what you put out there on social media sites reflects your self-esteem. Negative posts represent a lower self-esteem, which leads to lower mental energy. Try taking a social media break for a few weeks and see how you feel. See how much time you can spend on doing more positive things that push you further toward your goals of better health.

How much time do you spend watching television? Pick one or two shows that you enjoy and stick with those. Go to bed instead of binge watching shows on Netflix or Hulu. Think about the time that you will save.

MEAL PLANNING

Plan out the meals you will be preparing for the week. Make extra to have food for lunches already cooked and ready to go. Organize your grocery list so that you will only have to make one trip to the grocery store that week. This will solve the question, *What will I fix for dinner?*

Susan: *My grandmother opened up her own Rest Home when she was 60 years old. It was very uncommon for a woman to own her own business back in those days, but she went to California and trained under a rest home owner, and then came back home to open her own business. I would walk to her house after elementary school, which was a block from her rest home, and I so vividly remember her meal planning for the month. I was so curious how she went through the process of deciding what she would cook for the whole month. I'd ask her and she would say to me, "If I didn't have a plan, I might have the same thing too many times in a row and my people wouldn't like that. If I didn't have a plan, I wouldn't know what to buy at the grocery store and I would waste a lot of time and money." I remember her with her hand drawn calendar for the month, carefully placing what days of the week she would have chicken and what days she would have beef and so on. Then she would post a menu for the week on the wall for the people to see. I used that practice when I had my own family to look after. That lesson was so valuable when trying to decide what to fix for dinner and having ingredients on hand to cook the meal.*

Planning healthy meals helps to keep eating out during the week to a minimum. It saves time, money, and energy. You will never get healthy eating out. You will be able to control what goes into the recipes when you cook at home.

LACK OF FOOD CHOICES IN YOUR AREA

It is amazing that in this day and age, rural areas have little to no access to clean food choices. Organic vegetables and wild-caught, grass-fed meats are not available. If this is the case, check out food services that are available today. Fresh food is delivered straight to your door. Check out local co-ops in your area that offer organic foods grown locally. Go to the farmer's market. Many small farmers grow food sustainably without using pesticides but do not have the organic certification due to its expense.

SCHEDULE YOUR WORKOUTS

Put your workouts on your calendar just like you would any other appointment. Make them a priority. We often have good intentions, but when we look back at our week to see how many workouts we have done for the week, sometimes it's only one or at worst, life got in the way and we did none. Putting your workouts on your calendar and treating them as just as important as your other appointments is a step in the right direction towards your new body.

WORKING THROUGH PLATEAUS

Sometimes during your weight loss journey you might reach a plateau where you are not making progress in your weight loss. If and when this happens, look at your food journal or start journaling again. See if there is any mindless snacking. See if you are eating too much sugar. Make sure you are eating enough of the right foods.

Check out your sleep. Make sure you are getting eight hours of good sleep. Look at your sleep on the weekend. Try sticking to the same schedule you have during the week.

Check out your stress level. Has there been any additional stress that you are finding yourself facing? Remember to focus on breathing and meditation, and remind yourself that you are worth self-care.

FINDING A DOCTOR

Finding the right doctor that is willing to work with you and your health goals is important. Make sure your doctor knows how to properly test your thyroid and doesn't only rely on testing your TSH levels to determine your thyroid health. Search for naturopathic doctors or MDs who have extra training on natural ways to treat diseases. The number of doctors that are willing to learn a different approach to health is growing, as more and more people are looking for more natural ways to get healthy without reliance on medications.

EATING OUT

Everybody loves to eat out on occasion. When eating out, know what is in your area that will offer healthier choices. Pick out two or three restaurants that you know will offer food that is more appropriate for your new lifestyle and rotate between them. Read their menu on line and see what is available that will fit into your diet. Knowing beforehand prevents you from choosing based on what everyone else is ordering.

Skip on noodle dishes. Skip the bread before the meal and order a small house salad instead. Order steamed vegetable instead of ones sautéed in cream sauces. Ask you waiter to make substitutions for high calorie creamy sides. Try drinking a protein shake before dining out. Being really hungry prevents you from making the better choices.

PARTIES

Having a protein shake before a night out at a party will help with over eating as well. Choose the protein and vegetable appetizers and hors d'oeuvres over the carbohydrates. If you are going to drink alcohol, limit your consumption, staying with a glass of dry red wine. Drink water flavored with fruit. You can have fun without the extra calories.

NON-SUPPORTIVE PARTNER OR FAMILY MEMBERS

Making changes in lifestyle and diet is hard enough, but when you are also struggling with an unsupportive spouse or family members, your goals can seem like they are insurmountable. Your spouse may feel pressured that they are going to have to give up their favorite foods. He may make fun of your efforts to eat healthy. He may make negative comments about a new food you prepare for him. He may push the plate away and throw a tantrum about making him eat that food. All of this makes you feel that you are unworthy of fixing a meal that would benefit you and you must fix meals that keep him happy. You can't fix two different meals.

He may feel threatened by your wanting to change and that when you do change whether you will still see him as desirable. So what can you do to keep your goals on track?

- Have a heart-to-heart conversation about your goals and why you are trying to change your eating habits. Ask that he respect your decision to have better health. Tell him that you would like him to join you on your journey.
- Help him get involved with your journey by telling him what you need in order to make the changes possible. Like not bringing home the bags of cookies or chips. Even if your spouse does not want to join you on your journey, he may develop more empathy for you and even offer encouragement.
- Get him in the kitchen with you. Learn to cook together. Learn to remake his favorites in a healthier way that fits in with your new goals.
- If he is unwilling to support you, look into support groups or find a friend to help you on this journey. Remember you are worthy of doing this for yourself.

Family members that are unsupportive should be dealt with in a similar manner. Oftentimes, when you are trying to change, family members may feel that you are judging them for their choices. Have the conversation with them as well that you are doing this for your health and if they would like to join you on your journey, you'd love to get healthier as a big family. If they are unsupportive, it is a little easier than having to deal with an unsupportive spouse because you are not preparing dinner for them on a daily basis. Just stick to your goals and rise above distractions.

CHECK-INS

At the end of the week, check in with yourself. Evaluate how you did in meeting your goals for the week. Awareness of areas that need improvement keeps you moving toward your goals. Determine goals that were not met and determine ways that you will be able to meet them in the next week. Do you need to shift things around? What were your barriers? How can you carve out time to make sure you are able to meet your goals?

Aging

As you age your body responds differently to food and exercise than it did in your younger years. As you age, your hormone levels decline. This happens in both men and women. In women, levels of progesterone, estrogen, and testosterone start to decline. The amount of muscle may start to decline. Your body becomes less able to handle the amount of carbohydrates you once could eat. Long duration cardio will tend to stress the body more and will be less effective in helping you lose weight.

Add more weightlifting to your program. It helps to build muscle and strengthen your bones. Using weight machines at the gym may be better than using free weights to help you avoid injury.

Add more vegetables to your diet and maybe a little more lean protein, with less starchy carbohydrates. Play around until you determine your balance of nutrients. We are here to help, too.

Susan: *When I was younger, I was able to do very intense workouts. As I have gotten older, the thought of a long duration workout wears me out! Those types of workouts stress my adrenals a little more than they used to. I have modified my diet to get rid of extra sugar. I switched my workout routines to include high intensity interval training using weights, and I focus on weight lifting on other days. Working out has always been necessary for me to maintain a healthy weight. I usually get two to three HIIT workouts and one to two weight lifting workouts in a week. I think of this not as a punishment but rather as a reason to keep me on track to better health as I age. It's all in your perspective.*

Realizing and becoming aware of your obstacles is the first step in being able to persevere and push through blocks that are holding you back. Make up your mind that you are worth the effort that it takes to meet your goals. Become the *you* that you want to be. Don't let anything stop you!

CHAPTER 12
Marching Orders

"I've missed more than 9,000 shots in my career. I've lost almost 300 games. Twenty-six times I've been trusted to take the game-winning shot and missed. I've failed over and over and over again in my life. And that is why I succeed."

– Michael Jordan

on't look at having hypothyroidism as a dreaded disease as so many people do. Turn that thought around to see it as a reason to have a healthier lifestyle. See it as a way to help the others around you live their best life possible. When you focus on the negative, negative returns to you. Focusing on the positive brings positive to you. What you put out to the universe comes back to you multiplied. As my mother always says, *choose joy*! It is a choice. You decide how you want to react to a comment or a situation or to change. What is going to make you the happiest?

This book is a whole-body approach to healing the body and losing weight and keeping it off. Because it is never about just taking a pill or a supplement and expecting it to do miracles when you are living a toxic life. Just like the saying, you can't out-exercise a bad diet, you also can't out-supplement a bad lifestyle. This is a book that you can read and re-read to keep reminding yourself about natural ways of healing. Each time you read it, you will discover something new, something else that you can do to heal.

We've introduced you to Ella, a beautiful lady who feels defeated by her hypothyroidism and wants to know a better way of living in order to thrive and be there for her family.

We've told you about our stories and our struggles to get answers to why we developed hypothyroidism. Even though our struggles were numerous and felt insurmountable, we were able to get to the bottom of the problems and came out stronger in the process. We can look back and see that there is beauty in the struggle, and we have the opportunity and the obligation to spread the word about how we healed and continue to heal— and hopefully make a difference in someone's life.

We have talked about why the TSH test is not the best test to determine thyroid function. And that there are other reasons why you feel hypothyroid symptoms even when your tests are in the normal range. We've looked at inflammation as a root cause of disease and by reducing inflammation, the progression of disease stops. We've discussed why the health of the liver and the intestines play a vital role in thyroid function.

We have talked about starting with the brain and getting your thoughts on board before embarking on any journey to change. Building a vision board is helpful in getting your brain to see your life in the future and not dwelling on the past and present. We've given you tips on being more mindful and how to reduce stress by meditating.

We've examined about how diet is so important in healing the gut and the liver. No matter what diet you want to pursue, changing these things are a must in reducing inflammation and allowing the body to heal. Do these things first. They are the big rocks. We've given you action steps to help you begin to develop better eating habits.

We've talked about how our bodies are faced with toxins every day, and we have offered you ways to reduce your toxic burden to begin to clean up your internal environment.

We've looked at how stress adds fat to your waist line even though stress has no calories. We've given you ways to reduce stress and made suggestions for getting a better night's sleep. If you want to improve your ability to lose weight, make sure you are getting quality sleep. Sleep releases melatonin and human growth hormone both of which aid in weight loss.

We've studied the importance of exercise and ways to exercise so that you do not stress your adrenals. Exercise is necessary for a healthy life.

We've talked about how your genetic makeup might predispose you to developing hypothyroidism but developing hypothyroidism is more about your lifestyle, diet, and environment than genetics. This is true of most diseases.

We've looked at some obstacles you may face on your journey to becoming the new you and how you can overcome these and persevere.

We want to hear from you! Send us an email to let us know how you like the suggestions in our book and how they have helped you.

Our wish for you is that you are able to implement our suggestions and live your best life possible! If life sets you back, pick yourself up, dust yourself off, re-read our book and get back in the game! It's only failure if you stay down for the count.

Where you go from here is up to you. You decide that you are worth it! We have some things that will help you on your journey. See our Thank You page at the end of the book to grab those free gifts.

If you decide you need more guidance, we are here to help you! Fill out the questionnaire on our Thank You page to tell us more about you and how we can help!

Acknowledgments

SUSAN

I would like to thank my husband, Neal Tucker, for always being there for support no matter where my heart takes me. You've been my rock throughout our marriage and throughout this process of writing our book. Your support means the world to me.

I want to thank my sweet, sweet mother, Mary Lee Jones, who taught me the power of positive thinking even before *mindset* was a thing. Her moto is *choose joy*! She lives this every day of her life even when times are tough! She instilled in us that happiness is a choice and sometimes it takes effort, but it is still your choice. Another moto of hers is to *do what your heart tells you to do*. In writing this book, I'm doing what my heart is telling me to do, Mom!

To my father, Norman Jones, who taught me to never settle for anything less than the best that I could do. He taught me the value of self-evaluation. To always look back to see how you could have done things better. When I told him about Anna and I writing a book about hypothyroidism, he said, *Make it a best seller!* I wish you could have been here to see our dream become a reality, but I know you are watching us from heaven.

And last but not least, to my daughter Anna! Because of your struggles, I knew what to do when I was diagnosed with hypothyroidism. Who would have ever thought that there would be power in the struggle!

ANNA

To my husband, Clifton Austin, I can't thank you enough for always supporting and encouraging me in everything I do. My best friend, and my rock, I couldn't imagine doing life without you by my side every step of the way!

To my daughter, Alaya Austin, you are truly my reason for everything I do. You have given me the greatest gift in this world of being your mother. I want to inspire you to live a healthy, vibrant life and to fully chase your dreams and passions; this world is your oyster. You have an incredibly bright future ahead of you, baby girl, and I can't wait to continue to watch you grow!

And to my loving mother, Susan Tucker. I can't thank you enough for doing everything within your power to get to the root cause of my health issues as a child. For becoming a researcher and stopping at nothing to find out all you could on how to improve my health. Everything I know about nutrition, I have learned from you! I now understand a mother's love, with a daughter of my own, and how you would go to the ends of the earth for your children!

To the Morgan James Publishing team: Special thanks to David Hancock, CEO & Founder for believing in me and my message. To my Author Relations Manager, Margo Toulouse, thanks for making the process seamless and easy. Many more thanks to everyone else, but especially Jim Howard, Bethany Marshall, and Nickcole Watkins.

About the Authors

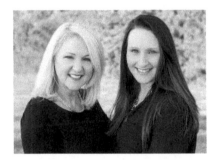

Susan Tucker and Anna Austin are a mother-daughter team who created their own health and wellness company, S & A Wellness Duo, to spread the word of health and wellness to their followers. They have an incredible, undeniable passion for health and fitness and natural approaches to healing the body.

Susan has a BS degree in biology and after 27 years of teaching high school sciences, retired to follow her passion, the healing power of nutrition. She graduated from the institute of

Integrative Nutrition and became a certified health coach. She helps her clients make better food and life style choices in order for them to live a more vibrant life. She lives with her husband, Neal, and enjoys spending time with her family and enjoying her wonderful grandchildren.

Anna has a BS degree in marketing and has worked designing websites and maintaining social media platforms for several companies for the past seven years. She decided to follow her passion and became a certified personal trainer and fitness instructor. Helping others has always been her passion. She helps to keep fitness challenging and enjoyable and feels that this is the key to lasting success and continued commitment. She lives with her husband, Austin, and their beautiful daughter, Alaya, and of course their fur baby, Bucc.

Together they are teaching what they have learned from their 19 years of getting to the root causes of thyroid disease so that those diagnosed with thyroid disorders can take back their lives –be able to lose weight and keep it off—and have energy and freedom from the symptoms of hypothyroidism.

Website: www.sandawellnessduo.com

Email: sandawellnessduo@gmail.com

Facebook: www.facebook.com/sandawellnessduo

Thank You

Thank you for inviting us to share with you our stories of healing! Our wish for you is that you live a life of abundance!

Do you feel like your hypothyroidism is sabotaging your efforts to lose weight, keep it off, and live a life full of energy and vitality? Are you ready to take charge of your own health and your own destiny? We are here to help you take back your vibrancy! If you are ready to change the future of your health, fill out the questionnaire and tell us your story.

www.sandawellnessduo.com/questionnaire

Contact us at sandawellnessduo@gmail.com and request information on certified pure, therapeutic grade essential oils and Nrf2 activation.

In Best Health,
Susan and Anna

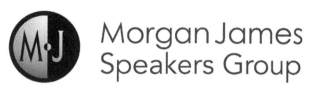

Morgan James
Speakers Group

www.TheMorganJamesSpeakersGroup.com

We connect Morgan James published
authors with live and online events
and audiences who will benefit
from their expertise.

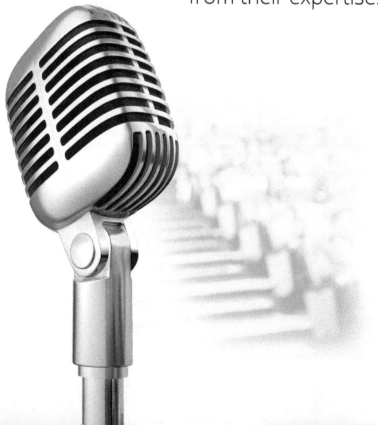

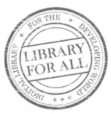

Morgan James makes all of our titles available
through the Library for All Charity Organization.

www.LibraryForAll.org